Bus

ADJUSTMENTS

ADJUSTMENTS
The Making of a Chiropractor

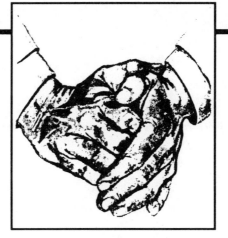

Vincent T. Joseph, D.C.
& Terry Cox-Joseph

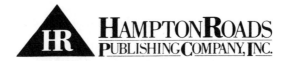

HAMPTON ROADS
PUBLISHING COMPANY, INC.

Copyright © 1993 by Terry Cox-Joseph and Vincent T. Joseph, D.C.

Cover design by Pat Smith
Cover painting by Terry Cox-Joseph

Hampton Roads Publishing Company, Inc.
891 Norfolk Square
Norfolk, VA 23502
Or call: (804)459-2453
    FAX: (804)455-8907

If you are unable to order this book from your local bookseller, you may order directly from the publisher. Call 1-800-766-8009, toll-free.

ISBN 1-878901-54-0

10 9 8 7 6 5 4 3 2 1

Printed on acid-free paper in the United States of America

Dedication

To the professors at Northwestern College of Chiropractic.
Thank you all.

Although the names and physical descriptions of the individuals in this book are altered to protect privacy, and many of the characters are composites, the stories, with all their humor, medical expertise, graphic detail and emotional turmoil, are true. In many cases, I'd like to relive the incidents because they were so rewarding and satisfying, particularly those where I helped an individual who was in despair or great physical pain. In addition, chiropractic, like other medical professions, offers those "Aha!" moments when some obscure textbook anecdote rises like a phoenix from the recesses of the subconscious mind and saves someone's life or alters the course of someone's life, and it is often those moments which mean the most to me. Other occurrences haunt me to this day. Some patients were virtually dead before they even crossed my threshold, offering me no chance at all to help them. Others simply didn't want to get well. And then there are the other health care professionals, employees, fax-machine salesmen, and family members whose knocks on the door changed my life forever. . .

To all of you, thank you, and I wish you good health.

Vincent T. Joseph, D.C.

PREFACE

My fascination with health care was spawned throughout the 1960s, '70s and '80s via TV shows like "Dr. Kildare," "Marcus Welby, M.D.," and "Quincy." Their plots held my interest because they successfully interwove the immediacy of life-and-death situations with the humanistic attitudes of caring physicians. It fascinated me that Marcus Welby would attend a patient's dance recital or Quincy would use up so much of his free time investigating cases that others were too lazy or incompetent to pursue on their own. Dr. Kildare, frankly, held no medical fascination for me. All I knew was that my older sisters mail-ordered pillow cases imprinted with his face and slept with him every night. Dr. Kildare was a sex symbol—ergo, doctors must be sexy.

My first encounter with the raw human aspect of being a doctor presented itself in the form of a visit with an emergency room physician who tried his best to be a decent human being but fell short of the mark simply because he followed protocol. The incident involved a childhood fall I took from a height of about five feet, where I did not break a single bone, but I bit off the end of my tongue. The doctor dutifully stitched up the offending body part and gave me a short sermon on how I was to stay away from solid foods which required much chewing and irritation, and by all means I was not to pull at the stitches or damage them in any way.

He then patted me on the shoulder and, as he had systematically done with hundreds of kids before, presented me with a red, cellophane-wrapped sucker. My raised eyebrows and pathetic expression caused him to blush furiously. I thanked him properly, of course.

That episode enlightened me to the fact that doctors are far from gods. They are individuals, operating within their scope of practice as best they can. It is this, the human side of health care, in addition to the Sherlock Holmes and Agatha Christie style investigations and intrigue that I find most fascinating.

What better way to merge the human and scientific aspects of health care than through chiropractic? Although chiropractic practices have been documented in ancient China and, later, Greece, as a bona fide profession in the U.S., chiropractic is only 100 years old. It is a budding, new and exciting field of health care and deserves to be brought forth beyond the rumors, innuendoes and fallacies that have smothered it for so many years. So many people can be helped in so many ways.

My husband can't write, by the way. I am his vehicle for written communication. Left to his own inventions, you would surely doze off after the third paragraph. But as an orator, he tells a great story. Enjoy!

Terry Cox-Joseph

INTRODUCTION

The smells of green tea and raw fish lingered in the air, giving me a feeling of contentment and fullness. We had just feasted on raw tuna, mackerel, yellowfish, shrimp and octopus, seaweed, rice, and a variety of pickled vegetables. The sake and Kiri beer were the perfect touch. That part surprised me; in America, I rarely drank—especially not beer. I couldn't even stand the smell.

But here, everything was different. I ate things that I would never dream of eating at home. I learned to enjoy vegetables that looked like something out of a science fiction movie. I actually relished biting into the tentacles of a tiny octopus.

I strove to express gratefulness and humility. At home, I was respected and, while I was kind, I was also aggressive and somewhat intolerant. Suddenly, I found myself totally dependent upon strangers for directions, train tickets, food and lodging. I knew enough about the culture to know that I was to remove my shoes when entering someone's home—and even the lobbies of some hotels. I learned to bow. I made certain never to offend people by slapping them on the back in that old American familiarity or touching their arms during conversation. I repeated *arigato*—"thank you"—so often, it was like a mantra.

What could I do to repay this family for welcoming Terry and me into their home and including us in their evening meal? How could I leave a little bit of America behind? What could I do to leave them with a smile and a feeling of comfort whenever they spotted an American?

Suddenly, one of the daughters reached around and rubbed her back. After sitting cross-legged on the floor for two hours, she'd become stiff and sore. She stretched her neck from side to side, her short black hair bobbing as she moved. She tried to straighten up. That was it!

"Let me show you something," I said. "I am a doctor, but I do not use drugs. I use my hands to heal. I fix bones that are out of place." Did they understand? Only two of them spoke any English, and it was broken, at best.

The girl nodded and walked over to me. I performed orthopedic and chiropractic tests for safety. The one test I always require is

Underberger's test—I asked her to close her eyes, tilt back her head, then raise both arms in front. At the same time, she was to rotate her head to the left for thirty seconds, then to the right. If one arm drops to the side, it's a positive sign for a vertebral artery insufficiency and I never perform any adjustments. An adjustment in that condition could cause a stroke and paralyze someone. Both of her arms remained raised. All of the other tests came out normal, as well. We were ready to go.

I told her to sit but made her face the back of the chair, straddling the seat. I stooped behind her as the rest of the family and a few friends—about ten people in all—huddled around to watch.

I motioned out her neck and spine by feeling each vertebra individually. Although there are tender spots, most people don't mind the process, and some even enjoy it. She had subluxations—tiny dislocations—in two spots in her neck and one spot in her lower back. With her fragile figure and petite stature, she was one of the easiest patients I'd ever palpated. She had an exceptionally long waist.

I stood before her and explained what I was about to do, demonstrating by cracking my knuckles loudly, then pointing to her neck. Giggles flittered across the room as the others watched. I then asked her to relax her neck, and I cradled her head in my palm. Slowly, I began to rock her head, then, when she seemed totally relaxed, I quickly made the adjustment. The sound it made startled everyone. Several people gasped. The girl's eyes flew open.

"Okay?" I asked, placing my hand on her shoulder. I wasn't worried about the physical familiarity, since she'd just allowed me to adjust her neck while her entire family looked on. She rubbed her neck and smiled, somewhat embarrassed. I knew that she'd never experienced anything like that before. "Let's do your lower back," I said. I brought two chairs together and stretched her out lengthwise on them. Placing her on her side, I adjusted her lower spine. The "pop" made everyone in the room break into laughter.

"Me next?" asked a young man, the girl's classmate.

"Me?" asked the girl's father.

Soon, everyone was gathering for an adjustment. "I hear of this," said one of the men, "but never see before. I want you to use your magic hands."

"Yes," echoed one of the sisters. "Do your magic on me."

SECTION I

"Youth is a blunder; manhood a struggle; old age a regret. "

Benjamin Disraeli, Earl of Beaconsfield

CHAPTER 1

"Doctors and lawyers must go to school for years and years, often with little sleep and with great sacrifice to their first wives."

Roy G. Blount, Jr.

"Why don't you want to be a veterinarian?" asked Terry, doing her best to encapsulate a lifetime decision into a ten-minute coffee-and-toast discussion before rushing off to work. I was groggy from having rolled into bed at 2 A.M. after a hard night as a waiter. I knew it was going to be a bad day when I discovered that my wife had used my plastic face razor to shave her armpits.

"Because animals don't talk to you. I need people."

"How about going to medical school? You love biology, you'd get to work on people all day long, and you'd make good money. You've been complaining about the restaurant so much lately that it seems like you'd really be much happier doing something else."

"I know that I've been thinking about my future, but I don't want to be a doctor. I don't want to see sick people all day. I don't want to give people drugs all day. And I don't like hospitals. I've spent enough time in them for my asthma."

"How about bioengineering? You could design body parts for people who've lost their limbs in wars and car accidents. You could design the next Bionic Woman."

"Because I'd have to go back to school and get a degree in engineering, and I don't want a degree in engineering."

"How about research? You're always coming up with ideas for great research projects. You could win a Nobel prize."

"Because I want someone to talk to all day. I'd go crazy doing research. The best projects take ten to twenty years and sometimes longer."

"Why don't you just do research on short-term projects at the University?"

"Because as a rookie they'd have me sweep the floors, feed the mice and sterilize test tubes."

She paused and gave me a quizzical, somewhat disgusted look. Her lips tightened over her teeth, tapering downward at the edges. "We've been married four years now. Why don't you know what you want to do?"

That kind of a comment was always good for a fight. Just because she knew what she wanted to be when she was five years old and never changed her mind didn't mean that the rest of the world had to follow suit. Colonel Sanders didn't start his Kentucky Fried Chicken empire until he turned sixty-five, and only then because he was insulted that his first Social Security check was society's implied opinion that he was now unworthy of a full-time job.

What was the rush? I was happily employed at Steak and Ale, meeting lots of people, making lots of tips and enjoying an occasional free meal. Someday I'd go back to school and the money I was making now could come in handy if we saved enough. Working as a waiter, I earned four times as much as I would have teaching or doing lab work with a biology degree. Maybe it was those tight black trousers I wore. Or the extra touches, like lighting the ladies' cigarettes for them. . .

But restaurant work was getting old. I didn't want to go into management, and being a waiter wasn't what I wanted to do for the rest of my life.

Why *not* be a doctor? I'd certainly been exposed to enough of them. I knew what I'd be in for. Memories of hot, stuffy afternoons spent in Dr. Murphy's office came flooding back.

"That wheezing has got to stop," he commanded sternly. I was barely twelve and would much rather have been playing baseball than sitting in this guy's office. I couldn't even respond to his conversation because I had to focus all my efforts on breathing.

"You've got to take allergy shots twice a week. That will help control your ragweed and pollen allergies, which, in turn, trigger your asthma attacks."

"Can't I come in just once a week?" I managed to rasp.

"Absolutely not. Twice a week at the very least. You're very lucky I don't have you coming in every day." I cringed.

My asthma was so bad that I had a heavy-duty household window air conditioner in my own room. My dad was able to deduct it on his taxes as a medical expense. I'd already been in the hospital three times that summer.

"If you don't continue taking these shots," he warned, leaning over to stare straight into my eyes so that I could see the broken blood vessels in the white parts and smell the stale tobacco on his breath, "you'll be dead by the time you're sixteen."

I gasped. His threat sent me into a brand new attack and I clawed at my chest with both hands in a vain attempt to ingest even the tiniest bit of air. A nurse whose ample midsection fit into her uniform only with extreme difficulty grabbed my left arm and jabbed a long needle into the triceps. I winced.

"Your lungs are shot," Murphy called after me. "No outdoor games. Stay in your room and read." He shook his head and disappeared into another treatment room.

Doctors. Their main goal in life was to scare you into health.

I continued to daydream, recalling the week before our wedding. Terry and I were enjoying the rides at a local theme park during the last open weekend that year. We stuffed ourselves with cotton candy, hot dogs and soda pop, and played dozens of games using darts, rings, pennies and squirt guns. We hadn't won a single stuffed animal but we didn't care. We laughed ourselves silly on the ferris wheel. We pretended we were spies, following each other menacingly on the excruciatingly slow kiddie train until the conductor kicked us off because we exceeded the weight limit. It was the kind of late summer weekend that those in love exploit to its fullest. As the hawkers at the stands sold their last few Cokes and Häagen Dazs bars, we walked hand in hand toward the entrance, the setting sun at our backs.

Suddenly, a strange whirring hum echoed through the trees. At first, we thought it was one of the rides overheating. But as the sound grew closer, not only could we hear the rumbling bass roar of an engine, but the penetrating, repetitive chop, chop of blades. Instantly, we knew it was a helicopter, even before we saw its hovering hulk break through the trees.

I'd been swatting at mosquitoes for the past several minutes. My arms were covered with them. They disappeared in an instant. I was perplexed.

"What's going on?" I asked, but I needn't have. Suddenly, a great wall of insecticide spread out before us. Sheets and sheets of the stuff blew in the breeze, dropping into the trees, onto the grass, skirting the food stands and rides. Why would an amusement park hire someone to spray just ten minutes before they closed?

"Oh no!" gasped Terry. "Your asthma! Run!" Coughing and gasping for air, we tore through the parking lot for the safety of the car, its rolled up windows a protective shield.

But it was too late. Already, my lungs were filled with fluid, and I knew I'd be lucky to make it back to Terry's house before passing out.

"Are you sure you want to take me home?" she asked, incredulously. "I'll take you to the hospital."

"No," I replied, salvaging my last vestige of machismo. "I'll take you home. I'll be all right."

She forgave me for not walking her to the door. It wouldn't have mattered—my sinuses were congested, my lungs were filled—how would I have managed to kiss her without passing out from lack of oxygen?

I showed up at the hospital every day that week in a valiant effort to make it to the altar in one piece. "Veddy, veddy sick," intoned a dark-complected female doctor with an Indian accent. "I never see anyvone so veddy, veddy sick." She began to wave her arms and pace back and forth. "Hospital. You go to hospital now before you die." Her voice lilted in a singsong manner, making her dire prediction seem comical.

Luckily, I had protected myself with a phalanx of groomsmen-to-be, who pelted her with protests.

"No, no, he's not that sick," said Bobby, my best man. "You should see him when he's really sick. He turns green."

Her eyes widened. "How could it be? Is not possible."

"He's getting married this week," offered another friend. "He can't go in the hospital."

"Just for two day," she said, rolling her r's.

"He's getting married in two days," countered Bobby. "Just give him a shot. Don't worry. We'll take care of him."

The withering look ejected by the doctor made us all shrink back into the shadows of the waiting room. Who did she think we were, anyway, roommates at Animal House? Cut us some slack, lady.

"I check," she said, still waving her arms and pacing back and forth with a little hop-step. We could see her consulting with a tall American in a white lab coat. They stood behind the corner in a small, makeshift lab. When the man shrugged his shoulders and rolled his eyes, we knew we were home free.

"I give you shot and many medication," she said as she walked back into the waiting area. "But you be sure to take all theez pills—you veddy, veddy sick mon."

There had to be another way. Another way to help people in pain, people who couldn't breathe, people who ached all over.

"I don't suppose you want to be a dentist?" Terry offered, jolting me back to the present. I shot her a warning glance and stared out the window.

"I used to go out with a guy whose dad was a chiropractor," she said. "They don't use drugs, but they're doctors."

Had she gone mad? Who did she take me for?

"What boyfriend?" I asked. Why did she have to start out the day like this?

"That guy I took graphic design with in art school. He wasn't a boyfriend, he was a friend. His dad is a chiropractor. It can't be all that bad—they're not rich, but I think that his mother gets to stay home, and they've got a house and a couple of cars. In other words, you won't starve to death, and you'd get to help sick people."

"I don't remember you going out with any guy in art school."
"That's beside the point. You haven't answered my question."
"So tell me about this guy."
"You're evading the issue."

It was like someone had snapped a picture of me while I was sleeping—the aftereffects of the flash were blinding. I couldn't see properly. I couldn't think. Art? Chiropractic? Boyfriend? Where was my morning coffee?

I called the chiropractic college and requested their admission requirements. I was sure that I could whip through the program in a year with straight A's. It would be like re-taking freshman biology. But the woman in the admissions office told me that even after five years at the University with a biology degree, I wasn't qualified. I had to go back to school in order to go back to school!

Not only that, but it was a four-year degree, and many of the courses required more hours than medical students had to take. The idea intrigued me. I toyed with the thought of wearing a lab coat and staring at a youngster, nose-to-nose, like Dr. Murphy had done so many years ago.

"Take my advice, Billy," I would warn him, in a deep, gravely voice. "Go outside and play. And don't come back in until it's dark. You need your exercise!"

CHAPTER 2

"Health nuts are going to feel stupid someday, lying in hospitals dying of nothing."

Redd Foxx

When I was seven years old, I had a paper route that forced me out of bed at 4:30 A.M. I forged my way through waist-high snow drifts, threw rocks at snarling mongrels, and tried to keep Mrs. Watkin's paper from getting wet because she always baked me cookies and gave me great tips.

The pouch I carried was designed for a 150-lb. adult man, so it was with great effort and noble intentions, not to mention a lean wallet, that I lugged the 40-lb. pouch diagonally across my body every day for ten years. I packed in as many bundles as I could carry at a time, and the weight was tremendous. Although I didn't know it at the time, the exercise helped my asthma; my lungs needed to be built up, and, although the smell of stale newsprint and fresh ink stung my nostrils and left imprints on my clothes and skin, I gave it my best shot.

After one excruciating morning, when ice caked the bundles and slick pavement threatened my every step, I hobbled into the kitchen, where my grandfather sat playing cards and sipping black coffee. My shoulders and back ached, and my head was cocked to the side. I felt like a scaled-down version of Quasimoto. My only thoughts were of bed and a heating pad.

"We'll take you to the doctor," Grandfather said. He threw on his coat and gloves and bundled me into the car. I took his word for it that I needed to see a doctor; he was my grandfather after all. Besides, he was a 6'4" foundry worker, all callouses and raw muscle, and he knew the difference between real pain and a whiny kid. I'd never been like this before.

The doctor's office was unremarkable in every way except for the fact that I could not detect the smell of rubbing alcohol anywhere. Doctors' offices always reeked of the stuff; it was their personal stamp of collective individuality. Restaurants smelled like grilled hamburgers; florist shops proffered wafts of greenery and moist soil; gas stations reeked of oil, gas, and cigarette smoke; doctors' offices smelled like alcohol.

At any rate, this doctor placed me on an exam table, checked my heart, felt around my neck, back and arms a bit, and then twisted my neck and shoved his hands into my back, and all of a sudden the pain was gone. Grandfather was right. I did need a doctor.

As I was stripping off my hat, coat, mittens and boots once again in my parents' kitchen, Grandfather explained that we'd just been to the doctor. Much to my surprise, Mom and Dad yelled at him. That was the first time I realized that some people didn't consider a chiropractor a "real" doctor. In fact, I'd never heard the word "chiropractor" mentioned at all until I got home.

"How could you do that?" they asked. "Chiropractors do all sorts of quack things with electronic healing—you could be electrocuted!" My mom had practical nurse training, so I figured she knew what she was talking about. I was getting pretty nervous. Had Grandfather done something wrong? We were in the dog house for sure.

"They're nothing but quacks and they take all your money!" I heard.

"But it was only two dollars," I said. "I saw Grandfather take it out of his wallet." My parents calmed down as I spoke. "You should have seen me! I couldn't even stand up. That stupid pouch was so heavy I could hardly walk, and my head was all twisted to the side and I looked like the Hunchback of Notre Dame. And now I'm perfect!"

It was a great testimonial. They shut up. And I never saw another chiropractor for fourteen years, until I enrolled in chiropractic college and, weeks later, ran into a chiropractor in the gym. He'd just opened up his first practice across the street and we spotted one another doing bench presses.

"So, you're starting chiropractic college this year? How often do you get adjusted?" Vance asked.

"Adjusted? I never get adjusted."

Dumbfounded understates the expression on his face. My ignorance hit me like a bolt from the sky. I was going to be a chiropractor and I hadn't been adjusted since grade school!

"Here, we'll use this bench," he told me. "I'll adjust you."

He examined my neck and spine in just a couple minutes, and, as he thrust the heels of his hands into my back, memories from the day at the doctor with Grandfather came flooding back. I'd forgotten how good it felt, how instantaneous the results, and how perfectly natural it seemed.

Vance soon became my personal chiropractor and never accepted any money I offered him. His contribution to my health and enthusiasm for chiropractic college were his rewards.

Months later, when I was a full-time student, I learned just what sort of quack sadistic electrical remedies chiropractors were supposedly foisting upon the public. What in the Dark Ages of the 1960s appeared to be quackery became commonplace and passé in the 1980s: electrical stimulation equipment such as low- and high-volt galvanic, ultrasound and Russian stim, equipment that many chiropractors and virtually all physical therapists use daily. I chuckled throughout my first electrical modality lab, remembering the fear my parents expressed so many years ago about "electronic healing." You've come a long way, baby.

Chapter 3

"But love is blind, and lovers cannot see the pretty follies that themselves commit."

William Shakespeare, *The Merchant of Venice*

You can't become a chiropractor overnight. It takes lots of college courses—in some cases, a full degree—and then four years of chiropractic college. Some universities even offer pre-chiropractic programs. The University of Minnesota offered a variety of degrees within the college of biological sciences that were perfect for pre-chiropractic students. Except that I didn't make up my mind about chiropractic until long after I'd received my undergrad degree, years after I was already married.

It didn't matter. As long as I was operating within the realm of science, I was content. Even during finals, when I lost sleep and operated on sheer adrenaline, I was happy to be doing what I liked doing best. And sometimes that led me into uncharted waters.

I have to backtrack chronologically to explain. It was the third week in April—the week from hell. Exams were rushing in from everywhere. Professors were demanding the impossible. University of Minnesota students were red-eyed, soggy-brained and, in a word, useless.

But not Vincent Joseph. A biochem undergrad, I whizzed through classes like a pro. Biochem was my forte. Yessiree, give me any chemical equation and I'd make the grade. I slept with the Kreb cycle under my pillow. I mixed cookie recipes using test tubes. Equations and formulas were second nature—I calculated intricate multi-leveled problems in my souped-up Pontiac, waiting for the red light to change. And the dank smell of gas from Bunsen burners and rubber tubing were like perfume to my nostrils.

I was never the dawdling type. There were things to do, places to go, and people to see. Youth had a tendency to do that. And that particular spring day, as usual, I was in a hurry and flew through my biochem lab a half hour before everyone else. It was a breeze.

And then came that little tug at my sleeve and heart strings, as the doe-eyed redhead next to me pleaded for help.

"I don't understand this lab," she said breathily, fluttering her eyelashes. Her cheeks glowed pink, complemented by the pastel pattern in her sweater. Her strawberry tresses flowed gently to her shoulders, moving as she moved. The closer she got, the better she looked—she was a living Clairol commercial, but there was nothing artificial about her.

She looked totally out of place in this lab. She belonged in interior decorating. Or English literature. Or art. I was still single, I rationalized. Although I was dating Terry, nothing said I couldn't enjoy lab work—and my lab partner. I had no way of knowing that one day I would marry Terry. This was the spring of my life. I was smart. I was smooth.

"How far have you gotten?" I asked. It was hard to concentrate on our conversation when her looks were so distracting. She was even wearing strawberry lip gloss; I could smell it. She was probably a model for all those nymphs in Walt Disney cartoons. Didn't I hear the "Dance of the Sugarplum Fairies" floating softly through the intercom system? Come to think of it, wasn't she in another one of my classes—calculus or something?

"Uh, I haven't started yet. Because I can't find the vass line." She squinted at the lab book. That's when I remembered that she wore glasses. They were wire rims, light-weight, perfect for her face; they added a bit of sophistication and a supreme look of intelligence. Not that she wasn't smart—she could run circles around me in calculus. But without the glasses, she was absolutely gorgeous. I just hadn't ever noticed before.

"The what?" I'd never heard of anything pronounced like that before.

"It says right here in the book—vass line." But I was too busy looking over my own completed lab work and notes to see what it was that she was pointing out. Suddenly, I forgot about her looks and started worrying about my own ass.

I blanched. The reference she was indicating was right at the beginning of the lab. Right before doing anything to the slides. How could I have missed such a peculiar item? I'd never heard of it before. I cracked open my book and proceeded to speed read the entire lab.

Nope. Nowhere to be found. Did I screw up? The invincible Vincent? Did I even do the right lab? Maybe I'd better ask someone. It was getting late. Only fifteen minutes left out of the hour lab. Would I have time to do the whole thing over again?

And, just as importantly, would I have time to help this helpless creature with her lab? Well, she was gorgeous. And she wasn't all that helpless, if calculus was any indication. This could prove worthwhile.

One more time. Just a look at the book. Was this elusive vass line a mathematical reference? Or something spatial—like upper and lower lines? Was it some sort of a baseline?

I asked her to point out the exact spot in the lab where it talked about this biochemical intricacy. I watched carefully this time as her finger guided me to the spot. There it was, as clear as could be: VASELINE. You were supposed to smear Vaseline on the slides to make them stick together!

I couldn't help myself; I groaned. Back to your first grade Basal Reader, eh, cutie? But when I blurted out "Vaseline!" the woman's eyes bugged out of their sockets in surprise. Her hands flew up to her face, and her cheeks practically caught fire.

"Ohmigod!" she cried. "I'm so embarrassed!"

I shook my head, staring at my feet and trying to hold back the belly laugh that was threatening to escape. "Do you think you can finish the lab by yourself?" I asked.

"My glasses," she said. "I left them at home. I am so-o-o embarrassed!"

"See you next class," I said, trying to distance myself before she started to sob. But that wasn't the only reason I made a hasty retreat. Because when she'd covered her face with her hands, I noticed a little gold band around the ring finger of her left hand. Oh well. I wasn't really fishing around, anyway. It really was Terry I was interested in.

CHAPTER 4

"Show me a sane man and I will cure him for you."

C.G. Jung

Psychology 101. There were over 1,000 students in the class. Can you imagine? How does one professor go about teaching that many students at once? Simple—he replicates himself. Our professor videotaped his lectures and played them during our large group meetings once a week in a huge auditorium.

In addition to our large group meetings, we were required to sign up as experimental subjects for ongoing research. One such research project in which I became involved was a two-credit course in computer surveying. It was a cinch. The other project was a little more complex.

A group of students, under the guidance of a facilitator, held a discussion group once a week on various topics. I wasn't quite sure about the purpose of this group in the beginning—the topics we discussed were nothing that were going to win anyone any prizes for originality.

But after a couple weeks, I began to see various personalities emerge. As a basic psychology student, I couldn't help but feel intrigued, because the two personalities that stood out the most were polar opposites. One student, Sam, a young looking, stocky black male, was quick to jump in and soothe any ruffled feathers that might have occurred while we were discussing controversial topics. The other was a square-jawed, hairy, olive-complected male whose attitude was about as apish as his appearance. Clyde was macho from the word "go" and certainly had no qualms letting anyone know about it.

After a point, Clyde had personally insulted everyone in the group at least once and had made everyone so angry that the majority of students wanted him kicked out. He was just too disruptive.

But just when things really started to get tough, Sam would jump in with a joke and a calming comment. Sam was a regular lifesaver. He always seemed to be in the right place at the right time. I ran into him the hallway once or twice and asked him to lunch, but our schedules conflicted no matter what I suggested, so I gave it up. I decided I'd just enjoy his company in the classroom and maybe I'd run into him again next semester.

At the end of our last class, the facilitator told us that the experiment had been successfully completed and thanked us for our time. Most of the students wandered off, but a couple of us asked what the experiment had been.

His answer shocked us: He was testing societal acceptance and avoidance of different personality types. Was it human nature to shun those who did not agree with everyone else's opinions? Who were argumentative? Crass? Angry? Rude?

Sam and Clyde weren't Psychology 101 students—they were graduate students and we were the experiment. Sam and Clyde were deliberately planted in the discussion group to force our reactions.

I felt betrayed. Particularly since I'd gotten to like Sam. What a creep! How could he do that to us?

I complained to the professor in charge of the research project. "This gives psychology a bad name," I said. "You're obtaining information through manipulation rather than general observation. It's easy enough—and scientifically valid—to study society at random when studying human behavior. Why this deceit?"

The professor was not swayed by my complaint. He shrugged his shoulders and said that graduate students were all allowed and encouraged to create and run their own experiments. His complicity in the matter seemed to have escaped him.

The experience soured me on psychology. I'd always been fascinated by the subject. My high school career profiles had always yielded test results that highlighted my skills and preference toward psychology. But when I read about the techniques used on prisoners of war and Jews in WWII, my fascination turned to revulsion. And then came those experiments by Stanley Milgram that I read about where participants were asked to administer electric shocks to victims on another side of a window to force them to answer a variety of questions. It was a Nazi-style test of allegiance.

There was no actual current, but some participants administering the shocks became obsessed with the ability to administer pain. A sad statement on human compassion, not to mention autonomy versus allegiance. The event was made into a TV movie starring William Shatner.

Psychology was rapidly losing its appeal for me. So when it came to large group meetings, the fact that I blended in with over 1,000 other students seemed apropos. Weren't we all simply gray matter waiting to be shaped by the powers that be?

A high school buddy of mine and I took the class together. It was somehow comforting to see Randy's familiar smile among that desolate sea of faces.

Both of our girlfriends were attending other colleges nearby, and, since we were all busy studying, it was extremely difficult to get together. Dates were for studying, not smooching in the back seat. We just couldn't afford the time. But we sure thought about it a lot!

One solution was for Terry and Lisa to visit us in class during the lunch hour. They could bring cheeseburgers and Cokes and we could sit in the back of the auditorium and munch during the lecture.

Years later, it now strikes me as exceedingly ironic that such a tactical error would occur in Psychology 101. There was absolutely no way that any work would get done during that lecture period. We were either eating, sharing French fries by chewing toward one another until our lips met or talking and giggling.

I feel that it's appropriate here to mention that I fell in love with Terry at first sight. I spotted her from across the room at a party. We all have our ideas of what the perfect woman is like, but, the instant I saw Terry, I knew that she was what I'd always been looking for. But preconceived notions can be very dangerous. You know all the old cliches: Don't judge a book by its cover. . .How did I know that her personality would match up to her looks?

My taste in dates was nothing if not predictable; they were all eggheads. Most of them wore glasses that had gone out of style twenty years ago. Their I.Q.s were well over 200. All we talked about was chemistry, calculus and quantum physics. I assumed they had kneecaps and elbows, but, since I had never seen them, I couldn't be sure. I blame this on my mother, who introduced me to the birds and bees at the tender age of ten by way of *Gray's Anatomy*. We all look the same when we're dissected, so what's the big deal, right?

Suffice to say that when I first spotted Terry, it was a first for me in many ways, not the least of which that I had finally been attracted to a woman solely because of her looks.

Her shoulder-length brown hair was naturally wavy and incredibly shiny. It bounced when she moved her head. Her nose was covered with freckles, and her grin was perfect enough for a toothpaste commercial.

After a brief introduction, I began to drill her on her resume. She'd been a member of National Honor Society in high school and was already on her way to a 4.0 in her freshman year of college. Unbelievable! Looks and brains in the same body! But my high would not last long; I discovered that, although she was highly intelligent, she also had a silly streak and an obnoxious laugh that could embarrass even the wildest exhibitionist. Once she got going, she just didn't know when to shut up.

Which leads me back to Psychology 101. After Terry and Lisa had shown up for a half-dozen classes, students nearby began to give us dirty looks and tried to silence us with noisy "Shhhhhhh" warnings. But it only got worse. And it escalated until, one day, Terry got a little clumsy with her ketchup packet. The contents flew through the air like an animated projectile and landed squarely on the pocket of my shirt. As I reached for a paper napkin to clean up the mess, she got the giggles so badly that tears welled up in her eyes and little animal-like squeaks emanated from her mouth. Ketchup matted her dark brown hair like clumps of blood, and mustard clung to her fingernails.

Randy's date thought the ketchup idea was great and decided to contribute. Red is such a cheerful color, don't you think? Before long, we were in the midst of an official food fight, and nearby students were issuing far more than polite "Shhhh" sounds.

But once you get going, you just can't turn it off like a switch. We giggled and giggled and began to roar and Randy fell off his chair and a couple students got up and moved and we finally all decided that it would be a good idea to leave.

Since the lecture had been such a hoot, the women wanted to come to the next one. Randy and I decided to skip it and just take them out to lunch. We were afraid that fellow psych students would be prepared with blowtorches and Dobermans.

We skipped the next class and opted for lunch at the local pizza parlor. And the next class. Pretty soon, I wasn't making any psych classes.

Inevitably, the time came for exams. It would be an understatement to say that I was unprepared. But I rationalized that the class has been worth it because I'd made my contribution to humanity: While I was ill prepared to write an essay on the differences between schizophrenia, hysteria and psychosis, I felt certain that my behavior had assisted the other students with first-hand knowledge of the disorders.

Luckily, university policy stated that students were allowed to drop one grade and retake any class they chose. I was out a few hundred dollars, but at least my GPA remained stable. My relationship, too, remained stable. I learned to keep it out of the classroom.

And, although I dropped Psychology 101, I know for a fact that I learned more than anyone else in that lecture hall.

CHAPTER 5

"It was so cold, I almost got married."

Shelley Winters

Three years was long enough. Long enough to kiss only between exams, double date whether we liked it or not and pretend that I wanted my freedom. It was time to tie the knot. So what if I hadn't graduated yet? I was only a quarter away. And besides, I would get a lot more studying done in the warmth of a cozy apartment instead of the God-forsaken frat house I was staying in. The front steps were crumbling, a couple of windows were broken, the linoleum on the stairs was cracked, and the entire building smelled like beer.

It was nicknamed Animal House, after the movie made famous by actor John Belushi. One night, the partying got so bad, I had to leave. The blaring music with its relentless bass rhythm I could handle, but the wall pounding and the sporadic outbursts of laughter and swearing wore me out. I threw down my books, laid my head on my pillow, locked my fingers behind my head, and stared up toward the top bunk, contemplating the difficulties I would have trying to step over everyone on my way down the stairs. Farrah Fawcett's beautiful eyes stared back at me, reassuring, silent. Her perfect body, poured into a skin-tight one-piece swim suit, beckoned me. But everyone knew that it was her hair that made her so phenomenal—layers and layers of golden curls, tendrils to run your fingers through, grab in your fists and inhale their heady perfume. Just look at that hair; it screamed "sex." Come to think of it, it *said* "sex"—it was actually spelled out in her hair. Why did I have to be so analytical, anyway? Did Farrah know that some photo retoucher had played with her hair? There—up past her ear, was the "S." Toward the crown was an "E." Near her forehead was the "X." It was as clear as could be.

I'd heard about subliminal advertising before. I'd been told that somebody came up with the idea that he could sell more snacks at movie theaters by flashing split-second photos on the screen. Eventually, a bunch of legislators got together and outlawed such mind games. But why did anyone have to do that with Farrah? She, of all people, needed no props. Aw, to heck with it. I threw my pencil at the poster taped to the cross-hatched wire supports on the bunk above me. I spent the night on the floor of a friend's apartment. It was uncomfortable, but at least it was quiet.

The next day, I returned to survey the damage at Animal House. The icing on the cake was the basement TV room that had been trashed. Beer cans littered the floor, the couch, the top of the TV. Some were crushed, some dented, some still half full, tipped sideways and slowly leaking onto the floor. Puddles of beer gelled on the linoleum. But what was that smell? It burned my nostrils, sweet but reeking of ammonia. That wasn't beer—it was urine! All over the floor, the couch, even the walls. Disgusting. Good thing I'd left when the going was good.

A week later, the mess was cleaned up—more or less—and I invited Terry to visit. I figured we could have a snack and work on some homework. I was running low on funds and really couldn't afford a dinner theater, much less the time it would take to go there. Terry agreed, and said she'd be right over. "I'm starved!" she said. She was always starved. I'd never dated anyone who ate as much as Terry. How she kept her size-2 figure was beyond me. Good genes, I guess.

When more than an hour passed, I began to worry. Had she forgotten? What if she were in an accident?

All of a sudden, I heard footsteps pounding up the stairs—not one set, but two, no—three. I couldn't tell—all I heard was pounding. Then men's voices made their way through the cracks in my door—laughing, cackling. "Wait," said one. "Hey, you," said another. "Get her!" shouted a third.

"Vince! *Hel-l-p-p!*"

Terry! As I flew off the chair at my study desk, she came tearing through the door. A chocolate shake flew through the air, crash landing on the floor. French fries ejected from a crumpled paper bag. Two bags of food, including hamburgers and ketchup packets, landed on my desk.

"What are you *doing?*" I shouted. She ducked behind me just as a 6'4" excuse for a human being came hurtling in the door after her. The stunned look on his face and the dull recognition in his eyes explained the whole thing. Another student, a mutant who had evidently been irradiated at birth on Three Mile Island, shoved his way past, then stared at me, dumb-struck.

"Oh," was all they managed to say.

I took a step forward, and they fell over themselves as they tried to maneuver the stairs. I recognized the bigger one as having eaten a beer bottle a few weeks ago on a dare. His lips and gums were still healing. I shivered as the memory of crunching glass between crushing molars ate away at my sensitivity. I slammed the door and locked it.

"What happened?"

"They were all sitting outside when I drove up. They started shouting things to me as I walked up. I almost turned around and went back, but by that time I was in the middle of it, and I had to step over them to go up the front steps. Then one of them said something about giving him some French fries, and another one tried to grab my arm. I think they were drunk."

"No kidding. Of course they're drunk."

"Anyway, then they really came after me. I was so scared, I just tore up the stairs and hoped that your door wasn't locked."

We began to sift through the remainder of the food. "There was a strawberry shake," Terry said apologetically, "but it fell. Do you want my chocolate shake?" She salvaged the remainder, wiping the drips on the edges with a napkin. "And there was another bag of fries, too. I guess they got their French fries after all. I can't believe a bunch of drunks would bother to chase me and scare the hell out of me just for a packet of French fries."

I turned to look at her, to study the expression on her face as she said that. Surely, she was kidding. She always did have a dry sense of humor. But her face was blank, her expression totally innocent. I was shocked. She couldn't possibly think that's all they were after.

"What's wrong?" she asked, staring back at me.

Before I could answer, her eye caught a piece of the Farrah Fawcett poster that had come loose from the bunk. She leaned over to look.

"No-o-o," she said, throwing me an outraged, bemused look. "I don't believe it."

She stretched herself out on my bed, locked her fingers behind her head just as I had a few nights ago, and stared at it. "You are so *sick!*" she said. "You are so weird. So this is the last thing you see at night before you go to sleep, huh?"

Embarrassed wasn't the word. Mortified, maybe. I know some guys who sleep with teddy bears. I knew a guy who drew a face on his pillow and hugged himself to sleep every night. I even know one who had a life-size, inflatable doll named Trixie. But that innocent poster caused me more trouble than I can ever say.

It was worth it, though. It made Terry forget all about her experience in the hallway, and that was worth all the heckling in the world to me.

That night was a turning point in my life. I wanted out. Out of Animal House. Out of dating. Yeah, the rent was only $50 a month, but I only had one little nerve left, and Animal House was threatening to rip it out of my skull. I'd often thought of marrying Terry. We'd talked about it many times. The idea was some hazy goal we'd never really set. Suddenly, it became my lifeline. After the experience tonight, I wondered what I would do without her. What was I waiting for? A mansion with forty-eight rooms?

That was the last "date" we ever had at Animal House. From then on, we ate out, went to movies, or had dinner with our parents. Terry even went out of her way to skirt the campus when she ran errands. No one believed how bad Animal House really was. That is, except for Terry.

Thinking about marriage sustained my last nerve throughout the summer. Terry was already renting an apartment with her best friend, and to say that I was jealous would be an understatement. She had laundry facilities. She had a dishwasher. A refrigerator. She had a balcony, and she'd invite me over to stretch out in lawn chairs and sip tall glasses of Coke. It was a respite from hours and hours of biochem and English lit and American history. Walking anywhere without a book under my arm made me feel absolutely naked.

September seemed the perfect time for a wedding. We avoided the typical June-bride syndrome and the Christmas rush. But a fall wedding would prove to be my undoing—because August and September are ragweed season in Minnesota, and asthmatics and ragweed are arch-enemies. And after running myself ragged all summer, overloaded with classes, working part time, and getting absolutely no sleep at Animal House, my asthma was preparing itself for a full military assault. Despite the pesticide I inhaled the week before the wedding, I survived. Barely.

My mother-in-law was highly complimentary during the reception. "My, you look so good tonight," she twittered, patting me on the side of the face. "I've never seen your cheeks so flushed—you're the blushing groom! It's so becoming."

I didn't have the heart to tell her that I was as high as a kite, having been pumped full of prednisone, epinephrine and champagne. My ears were ringing, and it wasn't from the sound of wedding bells. When would this whole thing get over with?

All I recall about the hotel suite was a silver bucket of champagne smack in the middle of the room when we walked in. That's the last thing I remember before I collapsed. The next thing I knew, Terry was soothing my forehead with a washcloth and pieces of glass. I could feel the blood dripping down my face!

"Why are you rubbing me with broken glass?" I asked her.

"Glass?" she said. "This is ice from the champagne bucket. You're delirious."

Deliriously happy. The happy honeymooners, off to a Caribbean cruise. . .and a miracle occurred: within hours after having set foot on the ship, my asthma and fever disappeared. I threw away my prescriptions and sucked the cool salt air into my lungs. Sea gulls disappeared in the distance as we sped off into the sunset, far away from the trappings of land. This was the life. I was going to move to the seaside and live on a boat with my beautiful wife.

If I could only find her. "Terry? Terry?" What was that green streak that just barely made it into the ladies room?

Terry later bragged that she spent her entire honeymoon in bed. The single pronoun generally escapes voyeuristic listeners in search of a juicy tidbit. I have to help them out and tell them that I spent our entire honeymoon fighting Hurricane David from the pool side, the shuffleboard deck, the midnight buffet and the gift shop—alone.

But that was all right. We got married for better or for worse. We just got the worst part over with first and saved the better part for later.

CHAPTER 6

"Cold nose, warm heart."

Snoopy

True love isn't about champagne and roses and chocolates and expensive restaurants. True love is getting your hands dirty and sweating and going hungry when you know there's something to transcend it all.

I was conducting an experiment on the St. Paul campus at the University of Minnesota. It involved changing the light sources and schedules of hundreds of philodendron plants. Since plant hormones are affected by light, altering the length of time between darkness and light would alter hormone production, thereby altering growth. Afterward, the plants would be chopped up into tiny bits, dropped into a solution and the results would be recorded. It was an exciting venture because its application in the Real World was so obvious. Farmers in the U.S., the Soviet Union and Scandinavian countries could farm the same crops, simply by referring to a chart.

My partner and I took on the project under the agreement that, since the plants had to be checked every four hours, we would split up the workload according to our class schedules. I'd check on the plants, which were temperature-controlled and monitored by computers for water and light, at noon, 4 P.M. and 8 P.M. My partner would do the same at midnight, 4 A.M. and 8 A.M.

It worked fine for a couple weeks. And then my partner wanted to take a couple days off at Christmas. Could I check the plants for her? No problem, just this once. I'd bring my wife along—how romantic!

Terry would keep me company. We'd make a date of it. It would be fun. And the whole thing would take less than forty-five minutes, since we lived so close.

But Terry wasn't convinced. Christmas Eve in Minnesota is not sip-iced-tea-and-watch-the-grass-grow kind of weather. It's the kind of weather that makes you shudder just to think about putting the key in the ignition while you wait for the slow, heavy chug, chug of the engine willing itself to turn over; that forces you to wear a scarf around your face because if you lick your lips, your saliva will freeze there and the next time you smile, you'll draw blood; that freezes the lakes so hard you can drive across them; that gives tinny voices and alien-like sounds to normally silent, inanimate objects like sidewalks and trees and walls.

So traipsing over to the U was not on my wife's priority list. But I convinced her—what an original way to bring in the New Year. And didn't she always want to see what it was I did all day at school?

Yes, she replied—in the daytime when the temperature is above zero.

I was thrilled. I gloated with pride, knowing that my research would help someone, somewhere else in the world someday. I was a dedicated scientist, monitoring a bold new experiment on Christmas Eve. The stockings were hung by the chimney with care, the tree glowed with multicolored lights, the smell of cocoa wafted through the air.

We drove up to the darkened facility just before both hands touched midnight. A fresh snow was falling, and my car imprinted the only tire tracks on the white blanket spread before us. We were alone on Christmas Eve, dedicated explorers, scientists, lovers.

Our footsteps echoed through the tiled hallways. An occasional light burned in various offices, forgotten by those who slept, dreaming of sugar plums and fairies.

The elevator door opened, and my jaw dropped. Another student! Someone else was working on Christmas Eve! We nodded to each other, brushing shoulders as he stood beside me.

My wife and I rode in silence as I began to rationalize the presence of another budding scientist on Christmas Eve. Then the doors slid open, revealing an entire building abuzz with activity. Dozens and dozens of lights glowed up and down the corridor. Voices hummed. Chairs scraped the floor. Scientists—students—professors—all working on Christmas Eve!

My ego was shattered.

Terry watched while I moved past the dozens of containers, checked the lights, put my little green urchins to bed, replaced a couple pens, restocked the paper and made a notation on the chart. It made me feel good, knowing that my wife was my best friend and partner and would follow me to the ends of the earth and praise me, no matter what.

"This is all you're doing?" she exclaimed suddenly. "Opening up little refrigerator doors and looking at these stupid plants? You're actually getting college credit for this? You have to pay money to take this class?" Her voice began to squeak. "I could do this at *home!*

Anyone could do *this!* What's the *point?* Do you want to see if you can speed up the growth? Slow it down? I can tell you the answer and save you all the effort of having to stay up all night on Christmas Eve when it's thirty-two degrees below zero, and you can pay *me* the money instead of the University!"

Sleep deprivation: It has a way of altering people's personalities—making them irrational and unforgiving. That's it! I'd do my next project on sleep deprivation.

SECTION II

*"Training is everything.   The peach was once a bitter almond;
cauliflower is nothing but cabbage with a college education."*

Mark Twain, *Pudd'nhead Wilson*

CHAPTER 7

They Tore Out My Heart and Stomped That Sucker Flat

Book Title, Lewis Grizzard

So this was it. I had my bachelor's degree in biology and I was going to be a chiropractor. I'd go back to school for four more years while Terry worked. I was going to be a chiropractor. I was going to be a doctor after all, but I wouldn't be pumping people full of drugs—I'd be saving them from fates worse than death! I was going to forge new heights in the health-care field, start my own talk show, open a string of clinics across the country and win a Nobel prize. No more undergrad work for me. I was into the hard-core stuff now.

"Why don't you want to be a *real* doctor?" my mother-in-law chided me. "Are you afraid?"

"Chiropractors are real doctors, Mom," my wife said, coming to my rescue. "Many of them are taught by M.D.s."

"Then why not just *be* an M.D.?"

"Because their philosophies are different. You always told me to marry a Jewish doctor. Well, Vince has a big nose and he's going to be a chiropractor. If it's good enough for me, it should be good enough for you. We could convert if it would make you feel better."

"Hey, nice to see yer back again!" exclaimed my uncle, smacking me on the back and laughing hysterically. "I'll bet going back to school can be a real pain in the neck—heh,heh. Aw, I know, you want me to get off your back, right?

"How many chiropractors does it take to change a light bulb?" he chortled. "One, but he'll have to go back for ten adjustments!"

It was just the beginning.

CHAPTER 8

"A vegetarian is a person who won't eat anything that can have children."

David Brenner

The smell that hits you when you walk into anatomy lab is nothing compared to the smell you take with you when you leave. It seeps into your nostrils like a living thing, clinging to pores and surface capillaries and mucous membranes. It attaches itself to your clothes. It hangs in the air like an invisible cloud, dampening your lungs with dewy pungence.

At night, it's not as spooky as it is lonely. You're literally in a room filled with people—but no one is there. Cold metal containers like something out of *Star Trek* glint halfheartedly, reflecting bits of light from the parking lot outside.

Our class immediately fell into a pecking order when faced with a dozen cadavers. The men became macho and the women wilted. Later, a few of the men wilted and the women became macha. Some of the students named their cadavers. That was verboten, according to school rules, but we did it anyway.

The cadaver I was assigned was an elderly white woman. To say she was not attractive was an understatement. She weighed about 300 pounds and hadn't washed her hair since she was forty-five.

We were never told what the cadavers had died from. We were not yet experienced in diagnosis. But it wasn't difficult to tell that this woman's weight was part of what killed her. We surmised that she'd been diabetic and may have had a stroke or heart attack.

During our first lab, we were to cut through the skin and fatty tissue in the back and work our way toward the spine. One of the reasons we started on the back was because it was less personal—less human— than the front, where you had to continually stare at the cadaver's face and hands. Those would come much later.

The first incision we made on our cadaver left a permanent incision on our psyches. Although this woman was dead, we all realized that she was a human being. She probably knew how to knit. Maybe she made little booties for her grandchildren. Maybe she loved soap operas and TV mail-order shows. Maybe her weakness was chocolate and she couldn't give it up even when her life depended on it.

But, at that very moment, this woman was a huge piece of flesh. And we were just then beginning to realize what a huge hunk of flesh that would turn out to be. Past the skin, we encountered an unbelievable amount of a substance that could best be described as scrambled eggs. We had all seen body parts dissected before—animal and human—but none of us had ever seen anything like this. We continued to cut, and remove, and cut, and remove, but, despite our efforts, the scrambled eggs seemed to be multiplying of their own will.

This cadaver contained so much fat—what is called adipose tissue—that we named her Adipose Addy.

Addy became a nightmare for our little group of four rookie health-care experts. We were supposed to have made it through the top layer of skin and fat in the first day. The next day we were to begin examining the muscles.

We tore away at Addy's fat tissue for three whole days. The labs were three hours long. We even came in after hours. That meant that we'd spent a minimum of nine hours just getting through the fat. We began to imagine just what it was that Addy ate to make herself so fat. Prime rib? Steak and mashed potatoes? Pizza? Sausages and scrambled eggs for breakfast, followed by a bratwurst for lunch and then a one-pound bag of potato chips for an afternoon snack?

Suddenly, food lost its appeal for every one of us. After working at Steak and Ale for four years, I had no desire to sink my teeth into their famous Steak and Bake dish, their prime rib or their sizzling filet mignon. I didn't care how much expertise had been necessary to create those elegant dishes, how much effort went into their preparation and appearance, which garnish was used with each entree, how much they cost, or what kind of wine was best with them.

I never wanted to be within smelling distance of anything even remotely resembling cholesterol. I did not want to die the way Addy did.

My wife was furious. "You promised me that when you went to chiropractic college you wouldn't turn out to be a health-food freak and now look at you—you won't even take me out for a pizza! Are you fat? Am I fat? If I were a cadaver, you could make it to my spine in one slice—and I eat pizza all the time! What is *with* you?!"

There was simply no way to explain it. She had to be shown.

At first, I balked at the idea of bringing my wife into the anatomy lab. It was against the rules. I'd have to sneak her in at night. Surely she'd leer and snicker and then, finally, gag and run, sobbing, out into the hallway. She'd make it into a regular circus show. These were real human beings we were working on. I hoped she understood that.

"It looks like something on a starship," she said, her voice echoing off the metal containers and tile walls. "How do you get these things open?"

I chose carefully, trying to remember which cadavers were most intact. I opened a container that held a thin, elderly black man. He'd hardly been touched.

"What happened to his skin?" she asked. "It's all gray."

"He's dead."

"You don't have to be sarcastic." She paused, staring. "May I touch him?"

I shrugged my shoulders. She reached out and touched his arm. She stared for several silent minutes at his hand. Then, suddenly, she jerked away and gasped.

"Veins! I can see veins! What's going on? I thought all the blood was supposed to be drained out!"

I was getting short tempered. "Those are tendons. Let's go."

"I don't want to go. I want to look at some more bodies. What did this man die from?"

"I don't know. We're not supposed to know."

"What are these little trays for alongside the bodies?"

"That's how we dispose of the parts we've finished with. Like the fat."

"I'll bet Addy's was overflowing." She grinned at me sideways.

We worked our way through a couple more bodies. I was careful to put everything back the way I'd found it. Finally, we left, walking down the hallway in silence. Terry sneezed.

"How can students work with that smell going all the way down the hallway? That would drive me crazy."

"The smell isn't in the hallway," I replied. "It's in your nose."

"It is not! It's all over the place."

"Then go outside and get some fresh air. You'll still be able to smell it out there. But it's not out there. It's in your nose. And on your clothes."

Outside, she inhaled deeply. "That's gross. What kind of a chemical is that? I'm going to have to go home and wash all my clothes."

I didn't say anything about Addy or my desire to give up red meat and other cholesterol-filled foods. I thought I'd let the seriousness of it sink in awhile.

A couple weeks later, we got in a new batch of bodies. Terry was dropping me off at the front door, where men unloaded containers filled with people who had no idea that they were about to make a donation to science. Behind us, students and faculty exited the rear door, going about their business.

"Look!" my wife suddenly exclaimed. "Chiropractors really can work miracles!" She pointed at the cadavers being brought inside. "You bring them in dead—" she then turned to face the back door and pointed at the students making their way down the hallway and out the door—"and they walk right out, as if nothing happened. It's a miracle!"

CHAPTER 9

"Who knows what evil lurks in the mind of man? Only the Shadow knows."

Radio show, debut 1930

At age eighteen, Candy was a so-so college student at the University of Minnesota. Although her love was for children and her goal was to teach, it seemed somehow that her real interests kept getting in the way—partying and talking on the phone. I'd known her for a couple of years and always anticipated her tall tales and bizarre sense of humor.

Her threshold for noise and consternation was high, but when it came to scary movies and ghost stories she was a basket case. She still bore emotional scars from childhood flashbacks of *Whatever Happened to Baby Jane?* and had an aversion to dolls that looked as though they might cackle in the dark behind her back.

The mere mention of a local murder (the last one, in which a local attorney seven houses away hired someone to kill his wife for the insurance, having taken place when she was an impressionable five-year-old) gave her goose bumps and created an involuntary muscle response that, when seated, caused her to lift her feet off the ground and wrap her arms around her knees.

Candy's boyfriend was well aware of this mental defect. And he was a bit of a defect himself. His idea of a fun-filled evening was to kiss Candy goodbye at the door to her apartment, then don a ski mask and sneak around back, where he'd lurk at the window, tapping and scratching. Every time she'd turn around, he'd duck. She never felt safe. Ever.

Candy waitressed at a Chinese restaurant, which provided her with great meals and more than her share of back pain. She was no stranger to chiropractic. She filled in the financial gaps selling Avon door-to-door.

The apartment building she headed for that memorable afternoon was right across the street, in a nice neighborhood. Mothers strolled the sidewalks with their babies, dogs barked, the mailman smiled and said hello.

But that was only a landlord's facade. Once inside the old brick building, the hallways were dark, the paint hadn't been touched up in years, the linoleum floor was cracked and badly in need of repair, and somebody's cat had claimed the far corner. Aside from the fact that the apartment building was so close to her own, Candy targeted it because it was one of the few in the neighborhood that allowed solicitors.

With a morning-after hangover from one of those little parties (you know, the kind where you start out with two friends and end up with half the campus in your kitchen, sloshing beer into your already half-dead potted plants), Candy wasn't so sure this was a good idea. But she needed the money. Besides, everyone thought it was so glamorous to sell Avon. The concept of all those women in the catalogs so prettily made up did, after all, provide a good incentive.

After three varied attempts at cold calls—one no answer, one slammed door and one grumpy old man—Candy was getting tired but thought she struck gold when a young man who looked like a dead ringer for Burt Reynolds cheerfully answered her knock. A little too cheerfully, she thought.

"Come on in," he said, smiling, gesturing warmly with his arm.

"Uh, I'm selling Avon. Is your wife home? Do you have a girlfriend?"

"I use Avon," he answered. She stood, dumbfounded, while he made her sales pitch for her.

"You sell men's colognes, shampoos, and specialty items during the holidays. I'd love to place an order. Come on in."

Candy's awe was replaced with horror. Her blue eyes widened as she saw what appeared to be a human skeleton in the shadows of the back bedroom. The theme from "Dark Shadows" flew into her head. She held fast to the door frame, goose bumps crawling across her flesh.

"Here—I'll pick up your order tomorrow." She threw the colorful booklet in his face, tripped over the cat in the hallway, and ran for the safety of her own apartment.

An Avon axe murderer? A pervert? After all, Minnesota was right next to Wisconsin, which had the unenviable status of being known nationwide for its mass murderers. First, it was the man after whom Hitchcock fashioned *Psycho*. Then, thirty years later, Jeffrey Dahmer. Maybe a few more nights waitressing would be safer. The warmth and glow of that little Chinese restaurant suddenly took on a stronger appeal.

But prodded by curiosity—and a negative checkbook balance—she returned the next day.

He was ready for her.

"I'm really sorry about yesterday," he said. "I bet you saw the skeleton in the back room." He smiled. Hmmm. No fangs, she thought. So far, so good. She gulped.

"I'm a chiropractic student at Northwestern. That's what I use when I'm doing my homework." When he smiled, he really did look like Burt Reynolds.

She nearly fainted with relief. "My brother-in-law goes there—Vincent Joseph."

"Hey, I know him," grinned the student. He placed a large order and became, thereafter, one of Candy's most loyal customers, much to her relief—emotionally and financially. Even though she still thought it was weird for someone to have a skeleton hanging in the living room. Or bedroom. Whatever.

Maybe he'd hand out some of her Avon booklets at the college. . .

Chapter 10

"Anyone who says he can see through women is missing a lot."

Groucho Marx

As a second-year student at Northwestern College of Chiropractic, I had survived the grueling mental exercises that are known for weeding out students who can't hack it and was on my way to the long, drawn out, nose-to-the-grindstone basics of becoming a doctor. My focus was becoming less and less aimed at rote memorization and test-taking and more and more at learning diagnosis and practicing chiropractic adjustments.

A chiropractic adjustment, also called joint manipulation, should not be confused with other forms of manipulation. For example, some physical therapists in some states are licensed to adjust the spine and neck by thrusting with their hands in one or two directions. But physical therapists are not trained in diagnosis, which is why most states require patients to visit a doctor first for diagnosis, then a therapist for treatment. What if there's a broken bone? You don't adjust broken bones. What if the joint pain is caused by cancer? Physical therapists are also not taught how to adjust every joint in every direction. Their adjustments, as are those of osteopaths, are designed to increase joint mobility, stretch muscles and break adhesions.

A chiropractic corrective adjustment is a precise, delicate maneuver. A good chiropractor can adjust each joint individually, in each direction. In other words, your best friend or sister may be able to pounce on your back with both hands and create that soothing "crunch" you love to hear, but the vertebra only moved in one direction because the thrust was only applied from one direction. In addition, your friend has no way of knowing which vertebra need adjusting—he's taking a shot in the dark. As a matter of fact, students who have difficulty locating out-of-joint areas and try to adjust anyway are said to use the "pound-and-pray method."

It takes months to learn the anatomy involved and develop the touch needed to find the problem area and adjust it. In some states, it's against the law for a medical doctor to perform chiropractic adjustments because of resulting pulled muscles and, in rare instances, the possibility of causing a stroke.

Lots of people confuse massage with chiropractic. "Oh, you're so lucky to be married to a chiropractor," people would tell my wife. "You get back rubs every day!" Sure, I know how to do massage, but I'm not specifically trained in it. An orthodontist knows how to clean teeth, yet he sticks to straightening them and hires a hygienist to do the cleaning. Massage can be relaxing or invigorating. It can help injuries heal faster. But massage deals with skin, muscles, tendons and ligaments. Chiropractic deals with the nervous system in addition to the musculoskeletal system. The beauty of chiropractic is how it helps the nervous system. Again, chiropractors are trained in diagnosis. Massage therapists are not.

At any rate, I needed practice. Lots of it. Practicing on fellow students during the day was great, but I was one of those students who had always excelled academically but couldn't seem to get the "touch" I needed. It seemed unfair that some students were born with it. I was just learning to find trigger points—little bundles of nerves and muscles that balled up into pea-shaped masses, embedded themselves in patients' muscles, and drove them crazy with pain. (Students have a lot of trigger points in the upper backs and shoulders because they're hunched over books all the time.) I had no trouble actually finding any of the vertebra. But each vertebra moves in six different directions, and if the patient was fat or quite muscular, it made the task at hand that much more difficult.

Practicing on my wife seemed the perfect solution to play catch-up. Her nickname was Lightweight, appropriate for her 5' 4" size-2 figure. I'd show up for class every morning just a little more secure, knowing I'd gotten in a few more minutes of practice. Even though the professors had warned students not to work on their spouses, hey, what was one little unsupervised adjustment? You didn't have to really do the adjustment—just set it up—feel around for a subluxation, take out the slack in the skin, place your hands in proper position.

Terry didn't mind, as long as she was convinced that I knew what I was doing. But every now and then, I'd pull a fast one on her. She never got hurt, but, well, she wasn't so sure. What if I invented a new neck adjustment to kill her and collect all the insurance money? Except that we didn't have an insurance policy.

Okay, she said, if you promise to give me a back rub afterward.

This new adjustment was really strange, I warned her. She had to be patient while I set it up. She already knew that I hated adjusting through jeans—I couldn't feel a thing. And Terry's jeans were always so tight that I couldn't get any hip rotation at all. So I had her unzip them. But that wasn't good enough. She had to take them all the way off—they were too restraining for side posture, the unique pretzel position.

Then I had her take off her sweater. Well, it was a thick cable knit. She could understand why that might be a problem for an inexperienced student. She was always so patient with me.

But the turtleneck underneath? It was below zero outside and drafty inside. Did she have to? Yes, I said. I had to learn to spot lesions and rashes and precancerous moles, too.

Then it was the hooks in the back of the bra that got in the way—those two nasty hooks rubbing right on her spine. Could be a potential problem there.

By the time she got to her underwear, the game was up. Wasn't there a movie called *Young Doctors in Love* or something based on this form of treatment?

She knew better than to check any of the textbooks the next day. Such adjustments didn't exist in any family-oriented books she was familiar with. Dr. Ruth might have something to say about it, though.

But the worst part—for Terry, at any rate—was that I couldn't resist telling a few friends at school the next day and the story flew through the hallways so fast that everyone wanted to try *that one* on their spouses.

Terry learned to dread school picnics and dances. "Hey, I heard you got a new adjustment. . ."

She'd get even. Someday.

CHAPTER 11

"Your picture tube is okay, but your cabinet has Dutch elm disease."

TV repairman in a Ziggy cartoon.

By my second year in chiropractic college, I had an ulcer, no friends outside of school, and hadn't bought any new clothes or eaten at a restaurant in two years. Unlike undergrad work, A's and B's in chiropractic college meant full-time studying. No outside jobs. I found that I could also excel in certain courses by becoming a teacher's assistant—a T.A. That required about seven and a half hours a week, in addition to the ten hours a day I was already spending at school.

Thank God I was already married. If I hadn't been, I would have been dropped by any sane girlfriend. What kind of fun is a guy who's always studying? But even my married friends were beginning to have problems. One was already going through a divorce. Two were fighting constantly. One couple wasn't speaking. Another friend was having an affair. Little did I know then that by the time we graduated and set up a practice, all but two of us would be divorced.

One of our professors once gave us a lecture on marriage and its place in our lives as students. "You probably all think that your spouses come first," he intoned, clasping his hands over his belly and staring down his nose over his glasses. "But while you're in school here, you're going to have to put your spouses on hold. You simply don't have the time to juggle it all. That means study in the evening instead of going to a movie. Study on the weekend instead of biking around the park and picnicking. Use the lab and library at school if you can't work at home. Eat in the cafeteria instead of your own kitchen. You have got to take this studying seriously because you are embarking on careers as doctors. Have you any concept of how important that is? Patients' health, even their very lives, lie in your hands. Five years down the line, you could misdiagnose a patient and kill him through negligence just because you decided to go to a movie with your spouse one night instead of studying. You could adjust someone's neck and forget the one chiropractic/orthopedic test that could have indicated a potential for stroke. How would that make you feel?

"Anyone who does not take chiropractic college seriously can just leave now. Get out. We don't need you. We don't want you."

His lecture spread through the halls like flames, eating away at hearts that burned with self-righteousness, souls that were driven to succeed, minds that craved answers before questions had been asked. Students argued in the halls, the cafeteria, in front of lockers, at the pool, in the gym, on the sidewalk. Some were incensed at the professor's audacity, his insensitivity, his callousness. Some waxed philosophical, taking it all in stride as yet one more thing on their list of "To Do's."

"He said *what?*" screamed Terry when I told her that night. "What a jerk! I'll bet he's not even married and he probably reads Nietzsche every night before he goes to bed!"

"I didn't say he was right," I argued. "I simply said he had a point. His point was that this isn't play time; it's serious business, and if we want to graduate we have to give this our best shot. Terry, you are the most important person in my life, but chiropractic college is the most important thing in my life. That means that we will spend less time together going out."

"Fine. I'll go out with my girlfriends. Sorry if I'm in your way, *Doctor!*"

It gave me much relief to know that other spouses had reacted the same way. But I knew they'd overreacted. We were all studying our tails off anyway; all that professor did was drive the point home. He'd just given voice to vague thoughts we'd all had at one time or another.

I had to admit that I needed a release of some kind, though. I'd cut back on my running, totally cut out any kind of clothes shopping or eating out, and spent virtually no time at all with Terry. I needed a way to unwind at night before I could even attempt to sleep. Sometimes I'd lay my head on the pillow, and so many thoughts raced through my mind, it was as if I was drugged or hallucinating. Voices, equations, bodies, books. . .I was too crazed to sleep but too exhausted to study.

My solution was to crash in front of the TV. It became a ritual, an electronic security blanket. "Quincy," "M*A*S*H," old-time movies and even an occasional "Gilligan's Island" episode kept me sane. I could watch human beings interact, problem-solve, tell jokes, argue, and go to war, and my only obligation was to lower the volume when Terry couldn't sleep. It was the one place in my life where my direct participation was not demanded.

Every now and then, Terry would wander into the living room in her nightgown, eyes squinting in the dim light, and chastise me for staying up so late. "It's 1 A.M. and you're always complaining about being tired," she said. "Why don't you come to bed?"

"I can't sleep," I said. "Leave me alone."

One night she stood in front of the TV and did a mock strip tease. I'm ashamed to admit that I was totally unmoved. The fact of the matter was, I was too exhausted to do anything but stare at her stupidly. Another night, she threw a bowl of popcorn at me. The kernels stayed on the floor for three days while we competed in a freeze-out. (I won.) Other nights, she ran to the bedroom in tears, rejected, vowing to torch the home of the professor who had brainwashed me with misogynistic ideas about marriage.

Something had to give, but I was at a loss for what sort of action to take. I didn't want my grades to fall, but I knew that my marriage was less than a model of perfection. I knew I shouldn't watch so much TV, but I didn't know how else to unwind at the end of the day.

"Unwind?" said Terry one night just before the clock struck twelve. "I don't care if you watch one or two shows. But once you sit down in front of the set, it's like you've plugged yourself into it. You're sick. You can't tear yourself away. It's like a disease. You're an addict."

I didn't think so. "It could be worse," I replied. "I could be out drinking like some of the students. I could be having an affair. I could be on drugs."

"You could be full of crap," she said, storming out of the room.

It got to the point that whenever I clicked on the TV, I braced myself for a full frontal assault. It was sort of like extra commercials; you hate them, but you put up with them because you really want to see the rest of the show.

I was getting an ulcer. My stomach ached. More than that, it burned. It kept me awake at night. No matter what I ate, it ate me first. School was getting me down. Terry was getting me down. I had nowhere to turn.

After a particularly harrowing day at school, I threw down my books on the dining room table, yanked a Coke from the fridge, and dragged myself into the living room for my evening dose of "M*A*S*H." It was like shooting up, but there was no crash when it was over, just a little commercial break and then another show.

But this time, something was wrong. Very, very wrong. There was the couch, just where it always was. I was holding my Coke in one hand and a bag of pretzels in the other, just like always. Had Terry rearranged the furniture? Something was missing. A chair? The stereo?

"Oh no!" I screamed. "The TV! What did you do with the TV?"

Terry sauntered into the room in her nightgown and stretched languorously, like a cat with nothing else to do but sun itself inside the porch door all day. She flicked a piece of hair out of her eyes, scratched her tummy lightly, and wiggled her toes, as if enjoying some little joke that I was not yet privy to.

"I got rid of it," she yawned.

"Where did you put it?" I ran to the bedroom. No TV. I threw open the door and ran through the parking lot out to her car. No TV. I ran back inside and peered inside the bathroom. Maybe she was playing some sick joke on me and had hidden the TV behind the shower curtain. "Where did you put it?" I yelled, desperate, panting. I was bereft. It was like she'd put the dog to sleep without my permission. Better yet, it was like she'd given one of our kids up for adoption and told me about it a week later. Never mind that we didn't have a dog or kids. It was a part of me! I couldn't live without it. What would I do?

"How could you do that?" I gasped. I was incredulous. Utterly astonished. She'd cut it out, severed it, cold turkey, no questions, no discussion.

"It was easy. I figured that something had to go—either our marriage or the TV. So I chose the TV."

"But you can bring it back, can't you? You didn't throw it away, did you?" I pictured the set sprawled half in, half out of the apartment trash container in the parking lot, its screen brutally smashed, the antenna bent in ways that no sensitive being should ever have to witness.

"No. I gave it away."

"Where?"

"What difference does it make? It's not coming back."

"I'll get it."

"Apparently you weren't listening when I told you that something had to go—either our marriage or the TV." She crossed her arms over her chest and her lips became nothing but a thin line.

I was beaten. Crushed. Drained. I threw myself onto the couch. I no longer had the appetite for my favorite Coke and pretzels. "Why do you always have to start fights," I whined. "Do you like living like this?"

"Yes, actually. This is the most we've spoken in weeks. It's not bad for a start."

She was serious. Dead serious.

I told everyone at school the next day. I needed a support group if I was going to make it through this traumatic period in my life. Their reactions were appropriate: shock and incense. But a couple of them had very sobering words of wisdom to offer me: Better the TV than the marriage, they said. Look at us—we're getting divorces. You're the lucky one.

Lucky? Me? Who were they kidding? I'll admit that I didn't exactly run home with a dozen roses and throw myself at Terry's feet that night, begging forgiveness. But we did have dinner together. It was kind of like starting all over again, in a quiet sort of way. When had she gotten that perm? And that new sweater? Yogurt ice cream? Strawberry yogurt? I didn't even know you could buy that stuff in the grocery store.

But Terry was still slowly steaming from months of abandonment. "I wonder what Hawkeye is doing now?" she snickered. "Don't you miss Hotlips? Or would you rather be watching 'Leave It To Beaver'? Or 'Star Trek'?"

I readied myself for the rush of adrenaline, the surge of anger, the verbal sparring that was sure to come. But do you know what? All of a sudden, I didn't care any more. I looked at the clock. The school library closed at 10 P.M., the signal to head for home. It was 10:30 and I'd already finished dinner and still had time to talk to Terry and do some homework. I had so much. . .I wasn't tired, but I wasn't as wired as I'd been lately. I'd actually gone to bed at 10:45 last night and it felt good.

Incredible, the things surgeons could do nowadays. I never knew how much a radical televisionectomy could do for your soul.

CHAPTER 12

"Friends share all things."

Pythagoras

Gynecology is not the first thing people think of when they think of chiropractic. It's another specialty altogether. But what if you've got a patient with back pain and no subluxations? The pain could be referring from an ovarian cyst, and you need to know whether to refer the patient. What if you're a chiropractor out in the boondocks and there's no OB/gynecologist within a seventy-five-mile radius?

My first gynecology exam was done on a dummy. I'm not referring to one of my classmates—I'm talking about a medical dummy like the kind you learned CPR on in grade school. A gynecology dummy is a little more complex, though. In certain areas.

It made it easy for us. We certainly couldn't hurt the thing. And we could probe for hours just looking and practicing and asking stupid questions and never have to worry. But the downside to using a dummy is precisely the same as the benefit—you can't hurt it. That's why we eventually practiced on a real person.

Linda was actually a very normal person. She wasn't an exhibitionist. She wasn't even a medical student. So we couldn't figure out why she would subject herself to constant gynecological exams by dozens of bumbling students all semester long. Sure, she got paid for it, but really, who would want to do that for a living?

When my turn came, I'll admit I was nervous. Linda was tall and slender, with ample hips, and, while she certainly didn't dress provocatively, often wearing a baggy sweatshirt and jeans, she exuded the kind of self-confidence that is, in itself, attractive. She was part Danish and part American Indian. Her honey-colored skin was flawless, and her eyes were a haunting green. We never found out what she did with her free time, but I pictured her camping out and hiking in the north woods, near Duluth. There was something about her that struck me as being tough underneath all that perfect skin.

I was scared to death I'd hurt her. But when I finished, she simply smiled at me and told me that I'd done a good job—at least, from what she could determine from her end. She told me that I was the gentlest of any of the students who had examined her. I glowed.

But I still wondered why she put herself through this. As part of our lab procedures, students practiced breast exams and hernia exams on one another, under the supervision of a professor. We didn't have to go out and hunt down patients when there were hundreds of available students wandering around. The idea was to learn to recognize healthy tissue and become exposed to a variety of body types. In addition, when someone you're used to sharing a Coke with in the cafeteria is probing away at your privates like a cattle rancher lassoing a wayward bison, you develop a heightened appreciation for just what it is you're putting your patients through.

It was rough doing those exams on one another. We were breaking each other down to minute body parts like lab specimens. It was demeaning. It was embarrassing. It was also one of the most important parts of my chiropractic education. I might never need to use any of these techniques throughout my lifetime of practice. But the information imparted through them was immeasurable. More than anything we learned about any medical procedure, we all learned something about friendship in that class. We were convinced that, after what we'd all gone through, we knew all there was to know about friendship.

Someone finally asked Linda why she submitted herself to gynecological exams all day when she could be out training golden retrievers or working at a health food store or teaching computer programming. Her answer stunned us into awed silence.

"My best friend died of cervical cancer," she replied. "I'd like to help educate as many students as I can so that other people won't have to lose their best friends—or their own lives."

CHAPTER 13

"You just gotta save Christianity, Richard! You gotta!"

Loretta Young, *The Crusades*, 1935

Jacob was one of those doctors who graduated in the bottom half of the class. As a matter of fact, he didn't graduate with his own class; he was held back two trimesters because he flunked embryology.

It wasn't that hard of a course. All it required was comprehending and few simple concepts and a lot of rote memorization. And that's what got Jacob into trouble.

To understand evolution, one need only to watch the process of transformation as a human egg is fertilized and takes on human form. The process, as anyone can see from photos, involves several stages which closely resemble amphibian embryos, complete with gills and a tail. Photos of a four-week-old human fetus, frog embryo and chicken embryo are difficult to tell apart for the first-time student.

Regardless of whether anyone in the class believed in the concept of evolution, they were required to memorize the course material and take the exams.

But not Jacob. Jacob called himself a Born-Again Christian. And evolution was antithetical to his beliefs. "So what?" we all asked him. "Just memorize it and then forget it after the exam. Besides that, the instructor never said you had to believe in evolution. All you have to do is memorize the names of the stages." But while some of the students tried to get Jacob to rationalize about the painlessness and expediency of rote memorization, there were those of us who knew that there was more to it than that.

Jacob believed that evolution was a plot designed by Satan. And, when it came to school, Jacob didn't know how to explain the fact that a fetus did not breathe air. But he refused to take an exam that simply stated that fact.

It took me awhile to realize that Jacob had his own brand of

Christianity. I had a hard time understanding Jacob. I had other friends who were Christians and they seemed at peace with their beliefs. But Jacob felt compelled to justify everything with belligerence and anger.

I loved embryology. And I believed in evolution. There's nothing to say that belief in God and evolution are antithetical. Albert Einstein was one of the greatest scientists who ever lived, and, with each new discovery he made, his faith in God increased.

The evidence of evolution was so obvious. . .That's why I loved science altogether, not to mention math—everything is logical and easy to follow. Now English grammar you can throw away, as far as I'm concerned. The people who write English books change the rules in every chapter. "*I* before *E* except after *C* except. . ." What's with all these exceptions? Give me my science.

At any rate, embryology is an important course for chiropractors because the formation of the spine is a fascinating and important process. It is there that the basic network of nerves is laid down. It is there that the connection between the brain and the rest of the body is formed. But Jacob would have none of it. He'd learn how to adjust the spine, but he would never understand why babies cannot hold up their heads or stand at birth or why their thumbs naturally face downward instead of toward the front. He'd never understand the origins of dermatones (tracing skin nerve roots), myotomes (tracing muscle nerve roots) and sclerotomes (tracing skeletal nerve roots), and, more importantly, how pain and numbness can be referred from one part of the body to another because of the patterns that are set down as an embryo.

For example, a patient can injure his neck at C-6 (the sixth cervical vertebra) and will experience numbness or pain in his thumb and first finger. Knowing how the dermatome, scleratome and myotome patterns work is essential for diagnosis. Even more, this type of knowledge enables you to build on future knowledge as new breakthroughs occur.

Jacob was so much of a Christian, as a matter of fact, that he would only treat Christians in his practice. That was always an entertaining topic for fellow students in the cafeteria. "What would you do if you saw a man bleeding in the middle of the street and he'd been hit by a car?" chided a woman who loved to call Jacob a male chauvinist pig right to his face.

"Help him, of course," came the reply.

"But what if you found out that man was a Jew?"

"Then I would not keep him as a permanent patient."

"What if you recognized him as a Jew before you went to help him in the middle of the street?"

Long pause. The philosophical debate of whether it was more important to honor the commitment of being a doctor or the commitment of being a Christian was being digested in Jacob's mind as his lunch digested in his gut.

"I'd help him because I'm a doctor."

"What if you knew he was a Satan worshiper?" teased one student. We all waited, eyes pivoted on Jacob. I heard someone snicker.

"I'd leave him there."

So much for Jacob's commitment to being a civilized human being. Not to mention his faith in his ability to convert someone. His ability to irritate other Christians, not to mention non-believers, was profound. The other Christians gave Jacob a wide berth. That left him with few friends and no study mates.

No one could understand why Jacob chose his particular brand of didacticism in the face of other compelling biblical examples. What about the Ten Commandments—all that stuff about loving your neighbor? What about the Golden Rule and doing unto others? What about "Whatsoever you do to the least of my brothers you do unto me?" Nonbelievers questioned other Christians in the class, hoping to be clued in, but the other Christians simply asked the nonbelievers not to lump them together with Jacob. They felt that his views reflected poorly on Christianity. That much was made perfectly clear.

Jacob was basically a likable guy. Red hair, broad shoulders, ruddy-cheeked with a touch of Irish and Welsh, he looked like the kind of guy you could smack on the back and share a few good jokes and a beer with. But, by his third year, Jacob's friendships were dwindling. Because he brought his wife to our dinner dances, a few curious couples sat with them, including Terry and me. I had tried on many occasions to befriend Jacob, but he'd built up such a strong wall around him that it was virtually impossible. So he became a curiosity. We found Sandy to be honest, charming, witty and gentle. She, too, called herself a Born-Again, but her personality was so divergent from Jacob's that everyone wondered what she saw in him. She was, in a word, sweet. We wondered if she knew that he ate alone in the cafeteria and studied alone in the library. I often saw him approach a group of students to chat, and then the group would suddenly dissolve, each going his own way in a big hurry.

And Jacob began to fall further and further behind in his studies.

While class after class passed through embryology with its references to evolution, students' minds, spirits and emotional maturity evolved as well. We learned to be a little more polite to Jacob—because Jacob didn't seem to be going too much of anywhere. And we learned to feel very sorry for him. He was always arguing. I'd never met such an angry person. Some people love to argue because it hones their debating skills, sharpens their wit and gives them a chance to be top dog. But Jacob was self-righteous to the point of no return; he argued simply because he was argumentative. He always ended up in the same spot. While we were engrossed by the subtleties of diagnosis and the chameleon-like qualities of the human body, and while we anxiously awaited our first chance to work on a real patient, to attempt our own "cures," Jacob was still arguing chapter and verse in the Bible, still slamming his fist on the lunchroom table, still staunchly defending each sentence in his holy book. His life held no wonder, no questions, no surprises—only solitary anger.

Jacob fell behind in his classes, and we rarely saw each other any more. Despite that, everyone knew who he was. And we all learned something from him that had little to do with religion specifically and much to do with philosophy overall: If you limit your studies and your practice because of laziness, ignorance or inability, you are also going to lose out on opportunities. Success comes to those who embrace life, not those who avoid it.

After falling two trimesters behind, Jacob transferred to another school and finally graduated. He knew few students in his graduating class. He set up practice in a small, all-white Midwestern town. I heard that he was sued for malpractice, lost the case and went out of business—all in less than a year.

And it all started with one little class in embryology.

Chapter 14

"When I make a mistake it's a beaut!"

Fiorello Henry La Guardia

Terry was feeling blue. She was tired all the time. She had headaches. Could she visit the student clinic and have someone look her over?

"I've got a better idea," I said. "I'm learning how to draw blood. Why don't you drive me to school tomorrow morning and I'll draw your blood and see what's up."

That sounded fine to her. She ate nothing after 9 P.M., and at 8 A.M. sharp we walked into the lab. I arranged all the equipment and Terry took a seat at a school desk—the kind with the desk top attached to one arm of the chair. She rolled up her sleeve and I wrapped a small piece of rubber tubing around her biceps to raise a vein.

"Can you hurry, please?" she asked as I puttered with the equipment. "I'm getting hungry." It was now 8:30.

I grabbed three vials for blood and inserted the needle into Terry's arm. It went in perfectly. She didn't even wince. I wiggled the needle around, but no blood appeared. "Ouch!" she cried. "What are you doing?"

"It worked the last time I did it," I said. "Let me try a different needle."

I found another needle in the drawer, and inserted it in the same spot. Perfect once again. But when I tried to actually draw the blood, nothing would come out. What was wrong? Was it the vacuum tube?

"Aren't you supposed to undo the knot you tied when you pull back on that thing?" Terry asked.

"Oh, yeah." I untied the rubber piece and watched it fall to the ground.

"You're really hurting me," she said. "I don't feel so good."

"Wait, I got a drop. There it goes." A quarter inch of dark red fluid filled the tube. I glowed. Then it stopped flowing. I pulled out the needle a little, wondering it I'd gone all the way through, but no more blood was to be seen.

"Low on blood today, huh?" I laughed. Terry wasn't laughing. She was pale and I could see the veins throbbing in her temples.

"Let me try another one," I said. "I think there's something wrong with this vacuum tube." I dug yet another needle and glass tube from the drawer, retied the rubber tubing around her biceps and prayed. Nothing.

"Untie the knot," Terry suggested.

It worked. For a second. I wiggled the needle and Terry cried out. "Stop it! You're hurting me! Just forget the whole thing!"

Well, I had enough blood for the tests, anyway. I'd just have to be a little more frugal with it. I labeled everything and placed the tubes in a rack, and when I turned back to Terry, she had her head between her legs. "Are you okay?" I asked, bending over and peeking underneath the desk top.

"No," she said. "I think I'm going to throw up. I'm dizzy. I thought you said you were good at this."

"I am. I don't know what happened."

After a half hour, Terry stood up to leave. Her head had cleared and nausea had been replaced by impatience and anger. "I have to go to work," she said, walking briskly toward the door.

"Wait," I said. "I'll walk you to the car."

As I tried to catch up, Terry marched down the hall, toward the cafeteria. As she ducked inside, no doubt to avail herself of the vending machines, another student stopped me and chatted briefly. I tore myself away and headed for the cafeteria.

Terry was talking with a couple students and their spouses. They looked concerned. One was patting her on the shoulder. What were they talking about? Me. I knew it. I'd never be able to face the class again. Terry yanked up her sleeve and exposed the most hideously bruised arm I'd ever seen. Had I done that? Oh my God. I felt so guilty. I stepped closer, and no one noticed my presence. All eyes were on Terry's arm.

"How did you do that?" gasped one of the spouses. It looked like Terry had been beaten and dragged, kicking and screaming, across miles of asphalt. Her skin, pale from months of snow and indoor seclusion, screamed with color.

"Vincent did it," she said. I could hear gasps and tongues clicking.

The woman who had been patting her on the shoulder was aghast. "What happened?" she said, quickly grabbing a cup of cheap coffee from the nearest vending machine. They all gestured toward the closest table.

"I had no idea you two were having problems," said one of the students. "You seemed like the perfect couple."

I could see Terry biting her cheeks to keep from grinning. So, that was the plan, was it? I was a wife beater.

"When did he do it?" someone asked.

"This morning."

"This morning? What happened?"

Terry paused dramatically, sighing, then looked toward the ceiling. She was thinking. Thinking hard. Finally, she came to a decision.

"He was practicing drawing blood." She smiled victoriously. I heaved a sigh of relief.

One student rolled her eyes. Another groaned. Another shook her head. Another sighed. All got up to leave. Terry was no longer soap-opera material.

She caught my eye as she headed for the door. "Nice move," I said. "You really had them going."

"Well, hey," she said, "it's not like you didn't do your part."

Later that day, I headed off a professor in lab and complained about what had happened to Terry. "Which equipment did you use?" he asked. I showed him the drawer. "Oh," he said, "that stuff is no good. We got in a bad batch. You're just supposed to use those on oranges. I've got the good ones over there." He pointed to another drawer.

She's going to kill me, I thought. She's just going to kill me.

CHAPTER 15

"It isn't easy being green."

Kermit the Frog

The student clinic at Northwestern College of Chiropractic held myriads of adventures for students. Patients from all avenues of life utilized the clinic's facilities and interns at a very good price. All students were required to practice in the clinic before they could graduate.

I really looked forward to it. I'd get to practice on *real* people, not my friends or a professor who corrected my every move. And the best part was that now I'd really get a chance to help someone and show the world how wonderful chiropractic is. It was a learning experience for everyone. We students learned to deal with human nature, more than anything.

When Mrs. Andersen brought in her ten-day-old infant, I was ready for the challenge. I glowed in my new lab coat. I fingered my stethoscope proudly.

It was the tiniest baby I had ever held, much less adjusted. I wasn't prepared for such a feeling of vulnerability. From head to toe, he barely reached the length of my arm from palm to elbow.

The infant's history was brief: He would only nurse on one side. He had been that way from birth. When Mrs. Andersen tried to nurse him on the other side, the infant would jerk his head around and cry out in pain. In all other aspects, he appeared normal.

Cute little thing. His skin was so soft, and his head bore just a few wisps of hair. And such wrinkled little hands! The nice part about adjusting babies, I thought, is that, because they're so tiny, you don't need a lot of strength. Plus, they are totally relaxed. There's nothing worse than a patient who tenses up at the instant you make the adjustment. And of course, babies may cry, but they don't argue with you. They just stare up at you with trusting, newborn eyes.

There was a definite subluxation in the baby's neck. And it was a cinch to adjust it. The mother wanted to try it out.

"Excuse me?"

"Let's see if it worked," she said. And with that, she unbuttoned her blouse and snuggled the baby up to her breast. What a happy baby! Nursing away, so contented, just as if there were never a problem at all. The little boy could now turn his head and nurse at either breast. I was pleased as punch. Wouldn't it be great if all problems could be solved that easily?

But being new at all this, I have to admit I was rattled. I was used to those mothers who discreetly tossed a little blanket over their shoulders so that no one knew what they were doing. This back-to-nature bit would take a bit of getting used to. I could see that right away.

But that was what this clinic experience was all about, right?

I had been raised in the city, insulated from cows and sheep and even kittens giving birth. My environment was devoid of those functions of nature that others take for granted. My learning came from books. I'd never been nursed; I'd come home from the hospital with a staph infection. I'd never seen any of my friend's brothers and sisters nursed, either. We'd been brought up in an age when it was fashionable to bottle feed. My books and films in classes all the way through college had prepared me for blood, broken bones, pain, dissection and a host of sexually-transmitted diseases, but nothing had prepared me for this simple act of nature. I was ill-prepared and immature. And angry. I felt cheated. But more than that, embarrassed.

If only I could keep from blushing. I could feel my cheeks burning—I was sure there was smoke emanating from the pores. And damn that Mrs. Andersen, she knew. She was smirking. Staring straight at me and biting her lip to keep from bursting out laughing.

I would much rather sweat out three days of finals than go through this. It never said anything in the college handbook about learning to stare people straight in the eye when your eyes had a mind of their own.

Then there was the day that I was assigned an eighty-two-year-old female who was suffering from low back pain. I took a history, which, at her age, was rather lengthy, performed a thorough exam which included a blood pressure check and heart sounds, and brought her into the x-ray room. She was petite and very alert. She had age spots the size of fifty-cent pieces, but her hands were steady and her eyes crystal clear.

As student interns, we were trained to provide female x-ray patients with a lead shield to protect their reproductive organs. I double checked the x-ray settings, pulled out a cassette, and set up for the shot. Then I draped the old woman in a very heavy lead gonadal shield. She looked a little concerned, but I told her that it was protocol.

She began to snicker. "But my dear," she said, her voice cracking and tinny in the little gray room, "I have nothing to protect. I'm eighty-two-years-old. Not only that, but I had a complete hysterectomy thirty-five years ago!"

It was even in her history. I remember reading it. I could feel my face go red, then yellow, then cadaverous white. I didn't know what to say. I think something came out of my mouth that sounded like "Uh, uh, uh. . ."

The old woman continued to laugh. It started out as a titter and then deepened, rising from her belly. She was roaring. "You just made my day, young man! I'll take that as a compliment!"

Lucky for me.

Chapter 16

"You can't depend on your eyes when your imagination is out of focus."

Mark Twain

Practicing at the student clinic took on a life of its own. Some days, I was sucked into its whirlwind activities like an ant. Other days, I thought I was God's gift to chiropractic.

I was just considering calling it quits for the day, when I was assigned a student from the business college across the street.

"A bunch of friends told me about chiropractic," he said. "Some guy named D.D. Palmer performed a miracle adjustment on a janitor named Harvey Lillard or something and restored his hearing instantly."

I told him that he was right on the money.

"I have a hearing problem and I know you can fix it."

Right, I thought. And I'm Oral Roberts. But I checked him out, and, sure enough, he had a whopper subluxation in his neck, just at the spot where the nerves going to the ear are located.

"I was playing soccer," the student continued, "and I got messed up. Somebody kicked me in the neck. Ever since then, my hearing has been shot."

Hmmmm, I thought. Maybe I could be the D.D. Palmer of the 1980s. The history matched the symptoms perfectly. One little cervical adjustment and we'd both be new men! Just think how fast that would spread through the hallways at school. Professors would invite me as a guest speaker for their first trimester students. I could write up the case history for a chiropractic journal. A newspaper reporter would pick it up from the journal and run it in the daily paper. This was getting exciting.

But I hadn't finished the exam yet. I used my otoscope to examine his ear. I wanted to make sure that eardrum was nice and healthy.

But I couldn't see the eardrum. I squinted. Maybe the battery was low in my otoscope. Maybe the bulb was burning out. Hell, I couldn't see a thing! What was in there—ear wax?

That was it—tons of earwax. I grabbed a bottle of peroxide and I swear I used half of it just on that one ear. I let it soak a while, and then I used a syringe to extract the contents. I'd seen a few dirty ears before, but I almost lost my cookies over this one. The bolus of wax I removed from that student's ear was a monster thing. I showed it to him. He was shocked. And also in possession of two perfectly healthy ears once again. The kick in the head was a red herring.

I wanted to adjust his neck, restore his hearing, and attain instant sainthood. I was disappointed. And I also felt like a heel. I mean, the main idea was that I'd helped the patient, right? I should be ashamed of myself.

Later that week, two students from the same college showed up at the clinic requesting that I clean their ears. The next week, three more showed up at the door. I'd earned a reputation, all right. I'd just have to lower my standards a bit.

CHAPTER 17

"Appearances often are deceiving."

Aesop

It was just a few minutes past noon and the clinic doctor, radiologist and all the other interns were out to lunch. The receptionist was reading a romance novel, and I was going over some of my old exam notes. When the old man showed up at the reception desk, I didn't even hear him come in until he cleared his throat. I showed him back to an exam room. He limped as he walked, favoring his right leg. His shoes, old and worn, made little scuffling sounds on the carpeting.

"What seems to be the problem?" I asked.

"I've been seein' chiropractors since I was a boy," he said, waving a gnarled hand that was well covered with age spots. "Been gettin' adjustments all my life. I know what chiropractic's all about. My hip's been botherin' me. I want an adjustment."

"Fine," I said. "But first, I have to give you a brief exam."

"I don't need an exam," he croaked. "I need an adjustment. My hip is bothering me. I don't need any of your pokin' and proddin'."

"Sir," I said, "this is a student clinic. It's clinic policy to examine every patient who walks in the front door. Your hip pain could be coming from a hip joint, or it could be coming from the spine. It could be muscular, or you could have arthritis. Whether I adjust you and how I adjust you depends on what turns up during the exam."

"Fine!" he shouted. "Get your damn exam over with."

I ran through a whole series of orthopedic tests—straight leg exam, leg drop, rotations—and nearly all of them showed signs of severe orthopedic problems. I was growing concerned. I repeated a few of the tests, glancing at my "cheat sheet"—the sheet of tests that we used to remind us in case we forgot any. My continuous glances didn't escape the old man's attention. I knew he thought I was taking too long.

"Sir," I began, "You're showing up with an awful lot of positive orthopedic signs. I'm concerned about it and I think you should be x-rayed."

"Jees-us," he snarled. "You need to do this for a class or somethin'? I don't have time to sit around and help you with your homework. I'm not doin' any x-rays. All I want is to have my hip adjusted." His eyes sparkled. He was full of spunk, this old man. He was angry, but it was the type of anger that was used to fend people off rather than spar good-naturedly.

He was making me mad. His manner was very forceful, and he was intimidating, but there was no way I was going to even try to obtain any joint mobility until I could see what was going on inside him.

I told him that.

"You're just treating me like a guinea pig," he complained. "You keep lookin' to your list to see what other tests you can practice on me. I'm not interested."

"Look," I said, trying another tactic, "if money is an issue, I'll give you the x-rays for free. I've finished all my x-ray credits so you can be guaranteed that I'm doing this for your benefit, not mine."

He shrugged his shoulders and sighed. I shot the films. I put him face down on an exam table and placed a hot pack on his lower back and an ice pack across his right hip. Knowing how impatient he was, I ran down the hall and processed the x-rays as fast as I could and threw them up on the viewbox.

What hung before me was a perfect shot of the lower spine and one half of a pelvis. I squinted, pulled off my glasses, wiped them with a Kleenex tissue, and put them back on.

There was no more than a thin shell of cartilage on that old man's right hip. The bone had been eaten away and the words for his disease were burned into my mind from dozens of tests I'd endured through the semesters. His hip had been totally destroyed by lytic metastasis— cancer. It was amazing that he could even walk.

I began to sweat. I loosened my tie. What was I going to tell this man? He'd just come in for a simple hip adjustment and now I had to tell him that he had cancer. How was I going to do it? I'd read all about cancer in books, I obviously knew how to diagnose it on x-ray, but how did I go about telling a real person that he was going to lose his leg—or worse?

I flipped on the overhead light and reached for the doorknob. My hand dropped and I found myself searching my pocket for a pen. I put the pen back in my pocket and reached for the doorknob again. My hand slipped over it, covered with sweat. How would I phrase it? Should I sit down next to him? Maybe I could bring him in here and show him the x-ray and let him see for himself.

I could hear the clock ticking on the far wall. He was probably ready to bite my head off by now. I was taking far too long. I grabbed a clipboard with my left hand, held my pen with my right hand, and marched out into the hallway, rehearsing the speech I was going to deliver to him.

I removed the ice pack and heating pad and helped him sit up on the exam table. I sat facing him from a chair. I stared at him, trying to decide what to say. The look on his face was resigned and very, very sad.

He could tell from the look on my face that what I had to say was very, very serious.

He spoke first. "So, you saw the cancer."

My jaw dropped. He knew! He knew all along!

He shook his head, and his countenance grew weary. His thick, bushy eyebrows hung over his eyes, blocking the light from above, blotting out any reflection. He stared at me with dark, blank pupils that only moments ago had challenged me, tried to stare me down, intimidate me. A long, deep sigh escaped his lips. I was his last hope. I would work a miracle. I'd adjust his hip, and make the pain go away like the chiropractor had done so many years ago when he was just a boy. I'd make it all go away.

I kept track of him, calling him every couple weeks. And then, one day, about two months later, no one answered the phone. On a hunch, I checked the morning's obituaries. His name was at the top of the list.

His was the first death I'd ever had to deal with as a doctor. I tore out the obit and stuffed it into my wallet. He knew that he was living on borrowed time. He was desperate when he came to see me. But that obituary would serve as a reminder for me to follow procedures just as I'd been taught. Some day, a patient would walk in my door and try the same thing. And I'd stick to my guns. It wouldn't matter whether the patient deliberately tried to talk me out of a proper diagnosis because of fear or ignorance. I vowed never to let the question, "What if?" haunt me after a patient walked out the door.

CHAPTER 18

"For fools rush in where angels fear to tread."

Alexander Pope

Because of our conflicting schedules, Terry and I often rendez-voused at home, at restaurants, or at our parents' homes. Terry drove her Toyota and I drove my little RX7. We seldom switched unless someone's car was in the shop.

Dinner that night had been delicious. I was filled with contentment and stuffed with chicken. Hot coffee warmed us as we donned our coats and scarves, slip-sliding down the steps, laughing, waving to one another. We hopped into our cars and headed for home. It was above zero for a change, and the roads were pretty clear. It was long past rush hour. We headed for the freeway, Terry in the lead. My mind was on graduation and what the future held for me. I'd been called "doctor" ever since I'd started back to school, I'd worn a lab coat, I'd worked in the student clinic; but the title wouldn't be real until I held that diploma in my hand. I could almost taste the title. I rolled it around on my tongue, savoring the essence.

I'd begun to sign personal checks using "Dr." before my name. I wanted the whole world to know. I'd worked hard for that title. I would make myself known wherever I went. Terry had been doing illustration and graphic design for four years now, barely making ends meet. Getting me out into a real clinic would change all that. We'd be successful. Wealthy.

I'd driven only a few blocks when I realized that I'd lost track of Terry. Oh, well. It was pretty unrealistic to think that we could make the eighteen miles home without getting separated.

Suddenly, as I entered the freeway, I was abruptly jerked from my reverie by a driver a quarter-mile ahead who started to spin out on the ice. A car to the right took a hasty exit, avoiding a collision. The car to the left veered off and continued on. By that time, I was on top of the scene. The car next to me sped up to work its way around the errant vehicle, but suddenly darted into my lane. I almost panicked when I saw brake lights. Fool! Where did these idiots get their licenses? I had no choice but to slam on my own brakes. I tried valiantly to pump the brakes, but to no avail. I started to spin out.

As my car did a 180-degree turn in the middle of the interstate, visions of graduation melted. I'd never graduate now, I thought, as I stared, open-mouthed, at the Cadillac that was headed straight for my door. I closed my eyes and braced myself for the impact. My ears were ringing. My mouth was dry. My fingers squeezed the last breath out of the steering wheel.

Nothing happened. I peeked out with one eye. The Cadillac was gone. I heaved a sigh of relief. Maybe I'd graduate after all. Maybe I could find out if I'd won a merit award at graduation. Maybe I'd make it home alive. Maybe I'd find out who started this whole thing and kill him before he killed anyone else. As my car skidded sideways, slowing to a precarious stop, facing the wrong way in the middle of the freeway, I swiveled my head to the left, craning my neck to get a good look at the idiot driver who had nearly gotten me killed and prevented me from graduating after four long years, and more importantly, carrying the title "Doctor." Whoever it was would pay.

My heart refused to pump. There was Terry, pulled over on the shoulder, wide-eyed with fear, open-mouthed with shock. Terry! Terry had started the whole thing! What was wrong with her? Was she trying to kill me? My own wife? After all these years of school, she wasn't even willing to give me a chance?

I straightened out my car before anyone else could cream me, then pulled ahead and blended in with the traffic. I could see her pulling out behind me, a tiny toy car in my rear-view mirror. My head pounded with leftover adrenaline.

Ten minutes later, I rolled into the parking lot at our apartment complex. I breathed a sigh of silent thanks that not a single car had been nicked, not a single person injured. I pushed open the door with trembling arms. Terry was parked in front of me and walked over to my car.

"A little slippery tonight, wouldn't you say?" she said, raising an eyebrow. Smart cracks came easily when she was under stress.

"I was trying to figure out who started the whole thing on the freeway," I replied. "I couldn't believe it was you!"

"I can't believe I almost killed you," she said, suddenly serious. "I just couldn't believe it."

We shuffled in the door, shivering. Had it gotten colder or was that the effect of the adrenaline?

"What happened?" I asked, still incredulous. Terry was a good driver. This whole thing was just a freak incident.

"I had just gotten on the freeway and I noticed that all the traffic was in the two right lanes. Nobody was in the left lane. It was completely empty. I wondered why. So I thought, hey, I'll go in the left lane. I wasn't even speeding! It was glare ice. Just solid ice. It totally caught me by surprise. I almost had heart failure. *That* explained why no one was in the left lane!"

"You gave everyone else heart failure, too," I said, but she didn't need a lecture any more than I felt like giving one. We were both exhausted. We both had headaches. It was still early, but we decided we'd had a long enough day and climbed into bed. Neither one of us spoke. Terry's head rested on my shoulder and after a few minutes I could hear her breath fall into familiar pattern of sleep.

"What-ifs" played tag with my brain cells. What if Terry was killed? Or what if I was killed and Terry was a widow? The sudden realization jolted my perspective: My death would have signified nothing except another freeway statistic. I was just another driver heading for home. What did it matter that I could be called "Doctor"? And now, alive and warm and well fed, what did it matter, still? Who really cared except for my immediate family?

Such humble musings deflated that ogre inside of me called Ego. I stared into the darkness, trying to console myself by fantasizing about my signature on checks, message pads, x-ray requests, legal transcripts. But the feeling of elation had passed. I knew now that I would no longer sign my checks "Doctor." Yes, that was my new identity, but I hadn't lost my old one. I just needed a close brush with death to make me remember who I really was.

CHAPTER 19

Mentor (men'ter, -tor), n. A wise and trusted counselor.

The Random House College Dictionary

One of the requirements for graduation at Northwestern was an externship anywhere in the country. Students were assigned the task of choosing a practicing chiropractor under whose tutelage they would work for one trimester. It was one of the most challenging and rewarding experiences of our educations. Unlike medical doctors, most chiropractors do not have the advantage of hands-on experience in a teaching hospital. Despite the United States Court of Appeals decision to let stand a lower court ruling in 1988 that the American Medical Association was guilty of professional containment and conspiracy, and that chiropractors were allowed to practice in hospitals, medical doctors and administrators have been slow to welcome chiropractors into the fold. The decision stated that chiropractors *may* practice in hospitals, not that hospitals *must* embrace them.

Although many chiropractors advertise for externs in the hopes of securing cheap labor, none of the doctors who advertised interested me. I had my eye on a chiropractor with an advanced degree in orthopedics who occasionally taught at our school. He was so full of energy and enthusiasm that he pinged off the walls. Although his practice was young, it was growing and I liked his philosophy. He was a born teacher. I sought him out.

. . .And was instantly rebuffed. He'd been burned before by externs and wasn't looking for anyone right now. He didn't need anyone stealing all his ideas and then setting up shop across the street.

I had no idea how to convince him that I had no intention of stealing anything, so I decided just to keep after him. Every time I ran into him, I popped the question. He probably thought I was the chiro-pest from hell, but I offered my services and told him that I admired his energy and that I had lots of energy and a lot to offer him.

He finally caved in, and my work as a "real" doctor began. I was shown the entire clinic operation and expected to carry my own load. I was also expected to obtain referrals. I was so excited, I could hardly contain myself.

Evidently, the feeling was mutual, because one trimester turned into six months, then a year, well after graduation, and I became a regular part of the show. I had my own following and brought new patients into the clinic on a regular basis. The skills I obtained and the lessons I learned would serve me well later in life, and, no matter how exhausted I was, I was overjoyed to jump out of bed each morning to face the day.

He became not just a mentor, but a friend, not to mention an acute source of entertainment and surprise. I'd be poring over a patient's files, frowning in concentration, and suddenly, behind the closed door of a treatment room, I'd hear him burst into song as he adjusted a patient. *LaLaLaLaLa-la la!* At first I was taken aback by his audacity, but later I became addicted to his uninhibited antics. I could do that, I thought. I broke into song once while adjusting someone's back, but my only response was a huge sigh and much shaking of the head. Although the patient was face down on the adjusting table, I could almost see him roll his eyes. Some folks can get away with that kind of thing. I learned I was not one of them. Maybe it's because I could never stay on key.

As doctors and colleagues, we worked together, went to restaurants together, partied together, attended seminars together, and my wife and I even babysat his daughter when he had to leave town for a weekend. We were nearly inseparable, causing Terry to feel pangs of jealously and possessiveness. Why wasn't I spending any time with her? Why was I putting this doctor on a pedestal? Wasn't this getting ridiculous?

What we didn't know then, but soon learned, was that Terry had time on her side. She had only to wait. And despite her complaints, when it came to patience and tolerance, Terry put dozens of biblical characters to shame.

As with so many relationships, I began to want something more. I found myself nitpicking this chiropractor's office procedures, the way he handled his patients, even the hours he kept. What once struck me as the ultimate in chiropractic care no longer enthralled me, and I began to question my motives, his purpose, and, every now and then, I dreaded going into work.

Sometimes an objective third party can offer a point of view that is so crystal clear, you feel like you've been hit over the head with a baseball bat. Or even an opinion from a semi-objective party, like Terry. So when she propped her feet on my knees for a foot rub, I listened to her as I massaged her tender soles.

"You've outgrown the place," she offered. "All the things you're complaining about are exactly the same things that you thought were great before. They're the same people and they're good people, but it's you who have changed. Maybe you need to start your own clinic."

"But he was the greatest teacher," I complained. "I learned so much from him."

"What you're saying is that you're disappointed in him because he has nothing more to offer you," Terry said. "And you feel guilty about that because you feel like you've betrayed him."

I didn't know what to say, so I just rubbed her feet and sighed.

"You told me that you thought he would be a great teacher and mentor for you, Vince. And you told me that he stated right at the beginning of your externship that the best teachers have the ability to teach their pupils to outgrow them. Instead of feeling guilty, you should be happy. You're doing exactly what he wanted you to do. You're giving him the ultimate compliment because you've proved that he is a great teacher. You needed this time to learn about office procedures and interacting with patients. Your first couple months of work, you saw four patients a day and were exhausted. Now you can see twenty-five. Look how far you've come! It's time for you to leave, Vince. You can open up your own practice and take in externs just like he did. And when they leave, don't you dare make them feel guilty, because it's what they're supposed to do. Just pass on what you learned and make the chiropractic field the best you can."

Where would I go? What would I do? There were so many chiropractors in the Twin Cities that I felt smothered and extraneous.

Fate must have heard my silent questions. It wasn't long before I knew exactly where I was going to go.

CHAPTER 20

"Thanks to the interstate system, it is now possible to travel from coast to coast without seeing anything."

Charles Kuralt

We'd been hibernating all weekend, the temperature hovering at 32 degrees below zero. We ventured out every four hours to start our cars, then gave up, removing the batteries so that we could warm them up inside the apartment and reinstall them later. The wind, howling like an arctic wolf through invisible cracks in the storm windows, stole any vestige of warmth under the shivering sun. The wind chill was 70 below.

We'd pigged out on popcorn and hot cocoa, beef stew and coffee, Oriental stir fry and hot tea. Every meal screamed for a scalding beverage to take our minds off the frozen wasteland we called home.

The newscaster broke into the middle of an "I Love Lucy" episode with a special announcement: The temperature had risen to 20 below! I was like a bird let out of a cage. "I'm going running," I announced to Terry. "It's warmed up!"

Running and weight-lifting had become my mainstays in chiropractic college, sustaining me physically when my mind threatened to desert me. The exercise expanded my lung capacity and increased my endurance. My asthma was virtually nonexistent except during ragweed season. Because anything even remotely resembling a life form froze solid during the winter months, all allergens disappeared. Despite the cold, winter became my favorite season. I could breathe. Ten miles a day was my lifeline.

I pulled on three pairs of socks, three pairs of sweat pants and a stretchy acrylic cap, covered my face with a scarf, put on two pair of mittens (gloves were useless because separating the fingers meant lost body heat) and covered the whole thing with a Gortex suit. I looked like I belonged in an outtake from a Woody Allen movie, but I didn't care. I was going running!

The first couple of blocks were heaven. The snow had crusted over and ice crystals glinted in the sun. Icicles hung from blackened tree branches, a contrast in opposites. An occasional surviving elm leaf, wizened and brown, tottered on the edge of a branch, clinging precariously, until a gust of wind snapped it off and sent it skittering across peaking drifts.

Lost in thought, I never saw the patch of ice in the middle of the sidewalk. A paper-thin layer of dusty snow had covered it, like a well designed hunting snare, there to trap an unwary critter. My right foot hit first, barely allowing me to follow through with the left foot and fall smack on my rear end on a cold, icy sidewalk. I could feel swirling currents of painfully frozen air even through my carefully layered clothing.

Composing myself as quickly as possible, I set off again, this time determined to keep a steady watch for potential pitfalls. As I left the protective barrier of our apartment complex and adjacent houses and headed for the lake nearby, I entered a clearing where the wind was allowed full play. A huge gust nearly knocked me over. It stung my forehead and brought tears to my eyes. The tears froze instantly and clung to my eyelashes. I tried to blink, but my eyelids threatened to freeze shut.

As I neared the second mile, my breathing began to grow labored. Even through the protective layers of wool across my face, the air bit through my lungs like tiny daggers deep in my chest. I swallowed, then moistened my lips. The moisture froze there, gluing the scarf to my already chapped lips. I was no longer the free spirit, running gaily across softly windswept fields of wildflowers. I was miserable. I hadn't even completed two miles and I was ready to turn back.

I ran for about five minutes with a mittened hand on top of the scarf, hoping it would act as a shield and allow my lips to thaw. It worked. My glasses began to steam up, my hand deflecting my warm breath upward.

Satisfied that I could make it a little longer, I pushed myself to run faster. Despite the cold, beads of perspiration began to form on my shoulders. Rivulets began to stream from my armpits, down my sides and between my shoulder blades. I could handle this. I needed the exercise.

Suddenly, another gust of icy air blasted me full in the face, and I heard a tiny "pop, pop." Blinking instinctively, I threw up my arms to protect my face. Some idiot had thrown a snowball and hit me in the face! But my face wasn't wet. And there was no one around. Not even a wayward deer.

Standing there in the bitter cold, I glanced around, feeling suddenly marooned and lonely. Where were my landmarks? Had the sun dipped behind a cloud? Then, suddenly it dawned on me: My glasses! My glasses had shattered! That wasn't any snowball—after I'd warmed up my face, the cold air had hit me so suddenly that the temperature change had shattered my glasses!

I took them off as carefully as possible, folding them into my pocket for the long journey home. I couldn't see a thing. I'd have to walk. Slowly. Carefully.

By the time I made it back to the apartment, I was aching with cold. I was beyond shivering. The rivulets of sweat had frozen to my skin and the outside of my Gortex was covered with a thin glaze of ice. I looked like a human snowman.

I pushed open the apartment door and had to squint to find my wife. As I walked across the floor, my bent knees made little crunching sounds as the snow cracked away from the fabric.

"That's it, Terry. We're moving. I can't stand it anymore." I held up my shattered glasses. "I can't live like this. We're moving south."

We spent the rest of the weekend studying a map of the U.S. With a yellow marker, we drew a horizontal line, dividing the country into north and south, like a pre-Civil War illustration. "Pick a spot," I told Terry magnanimously. "Any spot—below the line."

Six months later, we flew across Interstate 94 on four wheels in our quest for freedom and warmth. We ate our way across Wisconsin. Terry slept through the outskirts of Illinois and Indiana. I sang dirty limericks through Michigan. We talked about all our relatives behind their backs through Ohio. Gossiping about family made Terry homesick and she cried all the way through Pennsylvania. Maryland had a "welcome" sign that we missed because we blinked. Washington, D.C., took our breath away. We vowed to come back.

When we finally made it to Virginia, we were exhilarated and exhausted. Although we were thousands of miles from where we'd grown up, I felt a friendly pull here, a magnetism. Somehow, I felt like I'd come home. It was the perfect spot. We had the change of seasons. We had mountains. We had ocean. We had cardinals. We had magnolias, jonquils and dogwood. We had wildlife. We had an exploding economy.

We had no furniture. We had no jobs. But we had each other.

CHAPTER 21

"Knowledge must come from action; you can have no test which is not fanciful, save by trial."

Sophocles

I was nervous to the point of insomnia, but I was also shivering in delightful anticipation. I knew I could do it. It was time.

I'd spent the last four years preparing for the exams that faced me now. My home state exams that earned me my Doctor of Chiropractic and the right to practice in the state had been difficult, but I knew what to expect. The Minnesota board exams, provided by the state board of chiropractic, contained written questions specifically geared toward anything a chiropractor needed to know. In addition, x-rays were slapped on a viewbox for our scrutiny. Instructors acted as guinea pigs, judging our ability to adjust. It was four years of chiropractic college condensed into two days.

But because they ventured into unfamiliar territory, board exams in any other state involved a certain amount of knowledge and more than a certain amount of luck. The Virginia boards were no exception, but they were of exceptional interest because, unlike many other states which have their own chiropractic boards, Virginia's chiropractors are governed by the Board of Medicine. That skewed things even more than usual. Medical doctors have reciprocity in most states, which makes it easy for most M.D.s to move across the U.S. and set up practice anywhere without having to take state boards. Chiropractors have little reciprocity, and usually only in bordering states.

I'd studied for months before flying to Virginia, long before we actually moved, but, once there, I deliberately crammed for two days before the exams. I stayed up all night memorizing page after page of facts, statistics, diseases, diagnoses. I was operating on sheer adrenaline. I functioned well this way, I rationalized. It got me through four years of graduate school; it ought to work now.

I expected the typical pathology questions, chemistry queries, orthopedic tests. But as I plodded through the never-ending brain teasers, scratching away with my #2 pencil, the questions began to leave the ozone layer and venture into outer space.

Out of over 800 questions, only two dealt directly with chiropractic. The rest were pieces of obscure medical trivia, useless unless you thrived on TV game shows. In addition, throughout the test, the answers to many questions were directly determined by which textbook had been used as a reference. For example, one question asked about the dermatone pattern at the nipple. Whether it was T3 or T4 (the third or fourth thoracic vertebra) was determined by the textbook utilized. Luckily, I knew which textbook had been used, and which dermatone was preferred by the author.

"How does diet affect the testosterone level of Zucker Fat Rats?" one question read. They had to be kidding. What did Zucker Fat Rats have to do with chiropractic? And why should I care about their testosterone level? I certainly wasn't planning on feeding or treating sex-starved rats in my clinic.

As luck would have it, one of my long-term undergrad projects at the University of Minnesota involved work with Zucker Fat Rats. I knew the answer, but how that would make me eligible to pass the Virginia State Chiropractic Board Exams was beyond me.

The weekend I spent taking my board exams was the same weekend that would determine the futures of almost 100 newly graduated medical students, as well. They were testing just across the hallway. I struck up a conversation with a guy who looked about as beat as I was.

"Boy, those exams were rough," I ventured. "How did yours go?"

"Some parts were pretty bad, but I think I made it through all right," he replied, tossing some coins into a Coke machine.

"One of the hardest questions for me was naming the dozens of accessory bones in the foot," I said, shoving in my own set of coins and retrieving a Diet Coke.

"What?" the new M.D. said, guzzling half the can at once and making a sour face as he gulped.

"The accessory bones in the foot," I repeated. "I had to name them all."

He made another face. "I didn't even know they had names," he said, burping. He shook his head and walked away.

The Virginia State Medical Board exams are, according to most M.D.s, exceptionally relevant to their expertise. Plastic surgeons take a written exam and two days of oral exams relating directly to surgical case histories. Internists and family practitioners are grilled on diagnoses and a host of diseases. The chiropractic state board questions were akin to playing Trivial Pursuit, specifically designed to keep chiropractors out of the state.

I found out later that I was one of less than twenty chiropractors who had passed that set of board exams. Conversely, every single M.D. who'd tested across the hallway that day passed and went on to practice full time in the state.

Section III

"All the world's a stage, and all the men and women merely players."

William Shakespeare, *As You Like It*

CHAPTER 22

"He was outcast from life's feast."

James Joyce, *Dubliners*

In the Wild, Wild West, shopkeepers just starting out in business found a cheap spot on Main Street, hung out a shingle, and waited for the customers to stream in. There were no telephones, fax machines, TVs or radios to promote the business, so word of mouth was the most reliable—and often only—source.

The medical profession has long frowned upon advertising. Medical doctors who take on associates run proper business-card-style announcements in the local paper, as though announcing an elite nuptial agreement, never daring to mention the word "ad."

But they don't need ads, really. They have the old-boy network operating in their favor. They have massive hospitals filled with patients, many of whom have never been to a doctor before and find themselves suddenly under the care of one. They have years and years of reputation and mystique surrounding their profession.

Chiropractors have none of that. I was on my own. In a sense, I was the Urban Cowboy, hanging out a shingle, waiting for the line to form out front.

Without the least bit of business training or experience, I grabbed every business marketing book and tape I could lay hands on. I studied neighborhood after neighborhood before choosing a site, which, by the way, was heavily influenced by two Goliaths of modern society: 7-Eleven and McDonald's. Those two chains spend thousands of dollars on market research and demographics, and I was not about to let their hard work go by unnoticed. I set up my first clinic less than a mile from both businesses, banking on the premise that their research would determine where the growth in the community would lie.

They hit the target dead center.

Once my clinic was set up, I wasted no time running an ad for a chiropractic assistant. I knew exactly what I wanted: a middle-aged woman, whose kids were grown, who'd done a lot of volunteer work, who didn't have boyfriend problems. I needed someone who was outgoing and friendly, but nurturing, like a mother. Like my mother, actually. Of course, I couldn't say that in the ad. (Wanted: Dear Old Mom for chiropractic assistant position. Must type, understand computers, have good phone voice, proffer hugs when needed.)

Most of the applicants were recent high school graduates looking for their first jobs. They couldn't type, their handwriting was illegible, they snapped their gum during the interviews, and, worst of all, they had absolutely no idea what a chiropractor was. After explaining that no, I don't do surgery, and no, you don't have to know how to draw blood to work here, I decided to re-run the ad. I had obviously done something wrong.

As I was composing what I hoped would be the ultimate Help Wanted ad, the phone rang. It was a woman named Clara, who wanted to make an appointment for an interview. The fact that she even knew what a chiropractor did was encouraging, and I arranged the appointment for later that day. Something told me to hold off on placing the second ad.

Talk about gut instincts: Clara was the potential ultimate chiropractic assistant. I could almost see the halo around her head. She had worked for a dentist for three years, but had to move because her husband was in the military. Unfortunately, within a short time after the move, he filed for divorce. Even so, Clara decided to stay in town. She was originally from New Mexico, but loved the colonial flavor of Virginia and wanted to begin a new life here. She could type 80 words per minute and was familiar with both IBM-compatible and Apple computer systems. Her children were in high school, and she was looking for a job in the health-care field.

She was approaching fifty years old, and her laugh lines were exquisite. She had perfectly manicured nails and great taste in clothes. Her references checked out perfectly. I was set.

Those first days were so exciting, I could hardly contain myself. I was obsessed. Luckily, my enthusiasm was contagious. We typed up letters telling people who we were and what we did, obtained mailing lists and sent off the letters to thousands of residents. We took out a quarter page in the Yellow Pages, and even ran ads in the local newspaper.

It wasn't long before I realized that the newspaper ads were doing very little for me. After six months, I stopped running them. The direct-mail pieces provided me with a few patients. The Yellow Page ad provided me with yet a few more. But my most successful marketing tool was simply me and my big mouth. It was my enthusiasm that brought people in.

Not everyone shared my enthusiasm, however. I created a list of local orthopedic surgeons, thoracic surgeons, internists, neurologists and rheumatologists as potential referrals, and proceeded to phone their offices one by one.

"Good morning, this is Dr. Vincent Joseph," I said to the receptionist after dialing the first number. "I've just opened a clinic across the street and would like to set up a lunch appointment with Dr. Bonaparte."

"What did you say your name was? And what is your specialty?"

"I'm Dr. Vincent Joseph, a chiropractor."

Click.

That scenario was repeated, without exception, for two solid years. One office manager even told me that her office refused to accept chiropractic patients. I was outraged. Adrenaline surged through my body, and I almost dropped the phone. They couldn't turn away patients arbitrarily! Patients were human beings! What difference did it make where they came from? "You're so prejudiced, you probably don't take black patients, either!" I shouted, banging down the receiver. What was wrong with these people? Didn't they read the papers? Didn't they know that the Supreme Court had ruled that the American Medical Association was guilty of conspiracy against chiropractors and that medical doctors were now free to associate with chiropractors? Didn't people know that, in some parts of the country, chiropractors have hospital privileges? Weren't they the least bit curious as to what a chiropractor really did?

But I couldn't waste my time tearing my hair in frustration. I still had to choose medical doctors for referrals. Upon what could I base my decisions? I felt paralyzed. I had no choice but to grab a doctor out of the phone book whenever I had to refer someone. One day, I stopped by the hospital to pick up a patient's x-rays and began chatting with the nurse on duty. "Say, who's a good neurosurgeon?" I asked. She immediately shot back the name of a doctor who practiced at that hospital. "I'm surprised you haven't heard of him," she said.

Frankly, I was taken by surprise. I'd heard his name before all right—but not in a complimentary manner. I'd heard from several people that he was a jerk. I'd spoken to his staff, and they were definitely jerks. He had an "attitude." But so what? That didn't mean that he wasn't a good surgeon. This nurse must know what she's talking about, I reasoned, so I referred a couple patients. I had to really swallow my pride to do that because, of all the offices I'd called, his had been one of the rudest. But I had to remind myself that the patient came first.

As it turned out, that hospital nurse was right. He was a great surgeon. (Now, years later, he still has an attitude.) Meanwhile, I continued to attempt business lunches. Eventually, somebody had to have a free lunch hour to meet with the new guy in town.

And one day, it worked. I actually got through to the doctor. I'm sure that the only reason he accepted the invitation was due to his curiosity over this faceless chiropractor who kept his office filled with a steady stream of referrals.

After that, I only got hung up on every other call. My spirits were soaring. And then, one day, I was shocked to learn that my first patient of the day was a referral from a physician down the street.

Weeks later, I was even more shocked when the physician himself showed up with a sore back. "I think you can help me," he said. "Nobody else can."

CHAPTER 23

"They have ears but they hear not."

Psalm 135:17a

The very first patient who walked into my very first clinic was a mild-mannered, quiet accountant whose personality changed the instant he stepped into his Formula speed boat. He loved to rocket down the river like a teenager, spray flying in all directions, the wake spreading behind him. One particularly rough day, Cory and his wife were racing a friend and hadn't taken into account the severity of the waves. The sun was out, and that was all that mattered. Before Cory even knew what was happening, the boat crested a wave at peak speed, became airborne, then smacked down on the river like a truck hitting pavement. His wife broke her wrist as she was thrown sideways. Cory, who had been seated at the wheel, took the jolt in his lower spine and neck. He was incapacitated. His wife, despite her wrist, piloted the boat back to shore, where their friends called an ambulance.

Cory was x-rayed at the hospital and given pain pills and muscle relaxants. He had no broken bones and no cuts.

When he came to see me two days later, he brought his x-rays with him, and his foresight impressed me. I expected to have to call and pick them up myself. I treated him with kid gloves. I ushered him into the exam room, and spent an hour taking his history and doing orthopedic and chiropractic tests. I was going to make sure that this case was handled perfectly from start to finish. Not a single speck of dust would go unnoticed. Although I never for a moment doubted that, eventually, somebody had to walk through that front door, it was Cory who gave that nebulous "somebody" a name, and for that I will be forever grateful.

Cory told me that, immediately after the boat hit the wave, he felt pain in his lower back and then pain in the back of his head, so immediate that he thought he'd been shot. Any time he moved his head, the pain got worse, especially with sudden movement, like when someone called his name and he turned to look. He also said that his neck hurt all the way down between his shoulder blades, and his right lower back was hurting.

Cory's left arm and hand also hurt, he said, describing the pain as stabbing and shooting. He commented that the pain was more intense in his thumb. He curled his thumb to show me, and told me that his grasp was weak. He said he'd dropped a cup of coffee on himself this morning. Every now and then, he said, his left arm felt cold. The pain pills and muscle relaxants were worthless, he said, and he complained because they made him sleepy, but he was constantly nauseated and couldn't actually fall asleep.

After his exam, I placed ice packs on his neck and low back and moist heat on his mid-back. Then I ran interferential current for fifteen minutes for pain and swelling. Afterward, I stretched out the area manually and did some trigger point therapy. The muscles were already more relaxed, and I told him to come back the next day for a report of findings. I also gave him instructions for home care. By the next day, I knew that his spasms would have relaxed enough for me to adjust him.

I reviewed his x-rays again that night and wrote up his treatment plan. The next morning I was ready for him. I'd gone over his history, and I'd documented the results from his orthopedic tests.

"Cory," I said, showing him his neck x-rays, "you have no breaks here, but you have a couple cervical subluxations. You have a moderate straightening of the cervical lordosis with mild anterior cervical weight bearing. Your cervical flexion and extension exhibit adequate overall excursion and appropriate intersegmental progression of motion. You've also got a mild curvature of the cervical spine directed towards one side."

I paused, giving him a moment to ask any questions. He was staring intently at the view box, biting his lip. I then described the anatomy and physiology of the area, then switched films and continued: "As far as your lumbar spine is concerned, there is pelvic unleveling, low on the left, with a left lumbar listing. Some anterior weight bearing is seen in the lumbar spine. I noticed from the exam that you have a lumbar sprain/strain and lumbar subluxations and you also have thoracic sprain/strains and subluxations.

"To sum it up, you have cervicothoracic joint dysfunction syndrome with associated myofascitis resulting from an acute, traumatic, subluxation sprain and strain of the cervicothoracic spine caused by hypertension/hyperflexion injury induced by acceleration/deceleration trauma.

"Treatment will consist of spinal manipulative therapy, manual trigger point therapy, and adjunctive physical therapy including spasm relieving galvanic current, interferential current, and ice and moist heat."

I was so proud of myself. I'd explained every single detail without missing a beat. Nothing was left out. I smiled, more at myself than at Cory, and said, "Any questions?"

"Yeah," Cory replied. "What's wrong with me? Can you fix it?"

My jaw dropped. Was he deaf? Where had he been for the past fifteen minutes? I couldn't have gone into any more detail if I'd tried. What did he want from me?

"What's it going to take to fix me?" he repeated. "And how much is it going to cost?"

Detail. I'd gone into so much detail. I'd practically described the individual blood vessels for him. But as he stared at me expectantly, it suddenly dawned on me that detail was what lost it for him in the first place. He simply hadn't understood a word I'd said.

When I was a first-year student in chiropractic college, one of the first things we were taught was the K.I.S.S. formula: Keep It Simple, Stupid. Don't overload the patient's circuits with useless medical jargon.

I had just violated one of the cardinal rules of health care: I had just thrown an accountant head-first into a seven-foot mire of medical muck. I'd built up his confidence in me, sure, but I hadn't communicated with him. I was acting like an old-time doctor who intimidated his patients with medical jargon. No wonder he was looking at me like that. As far as he was concerned, I hadn't said anything at all.

"I can help you," I said this time. "You don't need surgery. You've got a couple spinal bones that are a little out of place and are irritating a nerve, and you've sprained a couple muscles. I'm going to push the bones back into place using chiropractic adjustments, and then I'm going to put an ice pack on the area, and alternate with moist heat. I'm also going to use some electrical equipment like we used yesterday. It will take about twenty minutes today, and then you can come back for six more visits. There's nothing here that indicates any permanent damage; you're actually very lucky. As far as the cost is concerned, Clara will be happy to assist you before you leave."

He was happy now. And even happier at the end of the week, when, after only three visits, his pain was greatly reduced, and I told him he could go back to work as long as he didn't try to lift anything. He was relieved because it was past the first of the year and he was gearing up for taxes and couldn't afford the time off from work.

On his last visit, Cory brought along a friend who had headaches and neck pain that he thought were brought on by leaning over a computer all day. That guy brought in his wife, and she brought in her hairdresser. I was on my way to the busy clinic I'd always dreamed of.

I just had to remember to keep it simple.

One night in the middle of February, my pager went off at 4:30 A.M. It was a woman who had been in a car accident but was sent home from the hospital with a clean bill of health. Suddenly, in the middle of the night, her injuries kicked in, not the least of which was a muscle spasm. I told her to meet me at the clinic.

It took me an hour to get her out of pain and relax the muscles. Somebody at the hospital had told her to heat her lower back, and the heat had made the swelling excruciating. I adjusted her, and she experienced instant relief. She was like a new person.

I yawned and looked at my watch: 5:30 A.M. Should I bother to go home? I'd just bought a new leather adjusting table, and the padding was cushiony but supportive. It looked so inviting. Maybe I could just relax for an hour or two right here, stretch out my legs a bit, rest my head. . .

The alarm on my wristwatch beeped me awake at 7:45. I didn't even remember closing my eyes, much less setting my alarm. It had only been a moment ago that I'd been working on a patient. I was groggy and my head pounded. But I could hear Clara bustling around, and I knew that it would only be a few minutes before the first patient came in. I tried to brush out the wrinkles in my shirt, ran my fingers through my hair, and walked up front.

Clara nearly jumped out of her skin. "Where did you come from?"

"I had a patient in the middle of the night and I fell asleep on my new adjusting table."

She broke out laughing and got me a cup of coffee.

It was one of our busiest days. I worked straight through my lunch hour and began to notice that the caffeine and adrenaline that had worked so well for me this morning were wearing off. I needed something to eat. And another cup of coffee. But a new patient came in, a white-haired woman who looked like she was in pain, and I didn't want to have her sitting in the reception area while I ran out for a sandwich, so I brought her back into the exam room.

Since Mrs. Stubbly was a new patient, she'd filled out our standard form, but I still needed some more information about her present condition, and whether it had been one of a series of injuries or whether it was something new.

"Start from the beginning," I told her, and as soon as I said it, I knew I'd made a mistake. I should have told her to give me more details on her present complaint. But I was tired; it had just slipped out of my mouth.

"Oh-h-h," she sighed, tilting back her head, a little smile playing at the corners of her lips. "I'm 65 years old, you know. I've got quite a bit to tell. I'll start from when I was 18. That's when I first noticed a little pain above my right hip. It happened on my first date, you know.

Now *that's* a story in itself. . ."

Her false teeth clicked repetitively, a metronome keeping rhythm for her words. Her voice droned on, a soft, melodic lullaby. "And then she said. . .and then I said. . .and then I remember. . ."

I have no idea how long I'd been asleep, but suddenly, a huge snort woke me up. It came from me. It was so loud, I scared myself. My chin had sagged onto my chest, and my pen had fallen to the floor. Mrs. Stubbly looked hurt, and not a little indignant. Staring me straight in the eye, she said, "Not a very exciting story, is it?"

"I had a patient at 4:30 in the morning," I said. "I'm really sorry—I haven't had much sleep. I need a cup of coffee. Will you excuse me?" She smiled sweetly, in the calm, understanding, incredibly patient way that only 65-year-old ladies can, and I tripped over myself on the way out the door.

That was undoubtedly the best cup of coffee I'd ever had, but I felt gulps of guilt catch at my throat as each swig burned its way down my gullet.

I returned to the exam room, coffee mug in hand, and proceeded to take the rest of Mrs. Stubbly's history. This time, I steered the conversation in a more appropriate direction, and I focused in on her, eliminating any other thoughts that tried to creep into my weary mind. I gave her 100 percent of my attention. WWIII could have broken out and I would still have finished her history. I try to do that with all my patients now.

I got Mrs. Stubbly out of pain within three visits, and she began walking a half mile every day on my recommendation. She came back once a month for adjustments. And I never, ever needed a cup of coffee to help me make it through her visits again.

CHAPTER 24

"Call me anything—just don't call me late for dinner."

Henny Youngman

Choirpractor. That's how the man pronounced it. He knew exactly what he was referring to. And he was convinced that he was pronouncing it correctly. After all, his uncle had been to one. And he'd seen the name in the phone book. Never mind that it sounded like a church elder who spent Saturday afternoons coaching cherub-faced young boys to eke out Christmas carols on key.

Not a doctor. A choirpractor. Doctors gave you drugs. Choirpractors moved your bones. They could even help your neck.

He wore a plaid lumberjack shirt and jeans and a John Deere cap. And he hung his thumbs in his front pants pockets. He was admiring the mural in the mall that spelled out "chiropractic" diagonally in gold letters. The background was a dark hunter green, whisked on to look like bold brush strokes. Tastefully painted, the mural simply stated that chiropractic cared for you, and featured my name and address beneath the word chiropractor.

I stood behind him, my arms filled with packages, admiring my new mural, excited about my new life, and listened to the conversation. I was curious about the outcome, and did my best to fade into the shadows.

"Why isn't there an 'r' at the end of the word?" asked the man. "It says choirpractor doesn't it?"

No, the artist explained, that's a noun to describe the person. Chiropractic is the system, the practice. It has a 'c' on the end of it.

"Are you the choirpractor?"

"No," the artist sighed, "I'm the artist. The doctor is working on patients today." She shot me the evil eye.

Education. That's what it's all about. It doesn't matter what they call you, as long as they show up at the door. Well, theoretically, anyway. Too many young doctors, fresh out of school, think that the world should bow down to their expertise and finesse. To call them anything less than "Doctor" is tantamount to throwing a tomato in their faces. But face it. Patients don't show up on doctors' doorsteps if they don't think there's some hope of getting better. That's the part that really counts.

"You're not really a doctor," fumed a squat, middle-aged man whose back pain resulted largely from the fact that he looked like he was about to give birth to a beach ball. "My doctor told me that chiropractors aren't real doctors. You can't do surgery."

"It's against our philosophy."

"Yeah, so where'd ya get your medical degree?"

"I don't have one. I have a chiropractic degree. I got it from a chiropractic college."

"You're not a real doctor. My doctor told me so. Show me your degree."

The only reason this man was in my office was because his wife was a very good patient of mine and, after hearing him complain about back pain for years, she talked him into coming in. He would much rather have been slugging a few beers down at the local bowling alley. I led him into my office.

The wall behind my desk sprouted every degree I'd ever gotten— two college degrees, a doctor of chiropractic, x-ray certification, board certification from two states, and many others. It had been my favorite, and final, gesture when setting up my very first chiropractic clinic. After the sawdust had settled, the carpet had been placed, the furniture had been delivered, and the fish tank filled, I spent a half-hour hammering picture hooks into the wall, hanging each diploma gently, carefully, lovingly.

The man stood in the middle of the office and gaped. "He told me you weren't a real doctor."

"Veterinarians don't go to medical school—they go to veterinary school. Dentists go to dental school. Chiropractors go to chiropractic college."

"Yeah, yeah," he said. "So just fix my back, doc. It's killin' me."

CHAPTER 25

"I can't get no satisfaction."

Mick Jagger

Michael showed up at my office because he was hurting from a car accident. He didn't come straight to the office, you understand—he took a circuitous route. He came all the way from Ireland, looking for work. Educated as an engineer, he was a pretty intelligent guy. But he couldn't find the work he was looking for. He took a position as maître d' at a restaurant in a posh local hotel. Soon afterward, he had the car accident.

Michael was well versed in the American way of medicine, because he'd been through it all.

First he paid a visit to a general practitioner, who prescribed painkillers and muscle relaxants and referred him to a physical therapist. The physical therapist used a hot pack on Michael's lower back, which Michael knew was wrong, because his muscles were in spasm and the heat would increase the swelling. Ultrasound made it even worse.

Dissatisfied, Michael complained to the general practitioner who had referred him. That doctor referred Michael out again—this time to a psychiatrist. Michael had emotional problems, the doctor said.

Michael told the doctor that since the birth of his daughter, who was now three years old, he and his wife could no longer conceive. He was impotent. Michael liked his woman. And he liked his drink. And he liked to show off his mellifluous Irish brogue by bursting into unrestrained song in the middle of restaurants or doctors' waiting rooms. Michael was happy-go-lucky, but he liked his luck to go his way, or no way at all. So Michael and his wife split up.

And now Michael, trained in engineering, was whiling away his days part time as a maître d'. Not surprisingly, he had financial woes.

The psychiatrist didn't think Michael was nuts. He just thought he had a lot of problems, not the least of which was back pain. He referred him to me. But Michael went back to his general practitioner instead. He told the doctor that his shrink had referred him to a chiropractor. The M.D. wasn't thrilled with the idea, but said, "If you've got to see a chiropractor, then go see Vincent Joseph."

I immediately took Michael off of hot-pack therapy and gave him ice packs. The swelling in his lower back went down immediately. He had subluxations in his lower spine and was adjusted several times. His back improved, but, despite his ebullient style, his spirits were still low. Often, he'd complain about his problems with his wife, telling me how much he missed her and how much it aggravated and scared him to be impotent.

One day, after a few weeks of treatments, Michael breezed into the clinic and, with an ear-to-ear grin, much to my surprise, announced that he was cured.

What about the pain? Still there. What about the money problems? Still there. I was concerned—what had happened? He seemed happy enough, but he was still so far from being well. He looked a little odd this morning. He'd always had an unusual swagger—sort of reminded me of an Irish Popeye the Sailor Man—but today he seemed particularly woozy. His nose was awfully red, too. Had he been drinking? Surely, knowing Michael, he'd stopped off at the bar to celebrate his good fortune, whatever it was. I pulled him aside into my office and asked him what he meant by "cured."

In response, Michael let out a huge belly laugh, slapped me on the back and fairly shouted that he'd gotten back together with his wife— and she was pregnant!

"Look!" he cried, unzipping his pants and exposing his erection to the world. "It works!"

"I'm very happy for you and your wife, Michael," I mumbled, doing my best to stare him straight in the eye.

With a grin that couldn't fail to infect even the snarliest Scrooge on the planet, he zipped himself up, slapped me on the back once more, and sauntered out into the reception area. He began offering authentic Irish soda bread to the staff and after he'd eaten his share, littering the carpet with crumbs, he danced out the door. No one ever saw him again, but they'll surely remember that big Cheshire cat grin on his face. And I'll never forget that big, well, never mind.

It wasn't long after my experience with Michael that Tessa became a new patient. She complained of low back pain and irregular periods. Her OB/GYN said that she wasn't ovulating, much to Tessa's dismay, because she badly wanted a baby. Tessa had gone through the first-thing-in-the-morning gamut of taking her temperature when she discovered that there was no temperature elevation to indicate ovulation.

Her next option was hormone therapy, but she wanted to try chiropractic first.

My exam on Tessa indicated a sacrum (the flat area just above the tailbone) that was cocked up so high that it was irritating the nerves in the area. That made perfect sense to me; it fit right in with what her OB/GYN had told her in regard to ovulation. And it also explained her back pain. I began a series of adjustments to Tessa's sacrum. I'd planned on a half dozen adjustments, but within just two visits Tessa told me that she was totally out of pain. Even so, I wanted to make sure that the area was back to normal, so I had her come in for two more adjustments.

A month later, Clara told me that Tessa had phoned with good news—she was pregnant! Tessa wanted to thank me for the adjustments—surely they had contributed to her good health and ability to conceive.

The months went by and I forgot entirely about Tessa until I ran into her at a party. She informed me that she'd had a healthy eight-pound girl and was working out at the gym, getting back in shape. By all accounts, Tessa was back in shape as far as I was concerned. She wore a tight-waisted cocktail dress and three-inch heels. She looked great, and I told her so.

As we were chatting about babies and exchanging compliments, Tessa became more animated, touching my arm often, throwing back her head in laughter. She loved being a mother. It was an answer to her prayers. Tessa's husband and a couple of friends wandered over, enticed by our laughter and repartee. Without a doubt, hers was the most provocative, if not amusing, testimonial I have ever received.

"I want to introduce you to my doctor," Tessa exclaimed suddenly. "He's the greatest! He's the one who got me pregnant!"

CHAPTER 26

"Now for good luck, cast an old shoe after me."

John Heywood

Mrs. Snider had been a patient on and off for several years. She knew a lot about chiropractic and wanted to know if I could help her son; he was having terrible headaches.

No problem, I said, bring him in.

George looked rotten. Beat. He had that pallor that people get when they're really in pain. He was glassy-eyed and his skin was damp.

He showed up on a Monday and said that he'd had headaches all weekend. He told me that he'd been playing volleyball Saturday when he'd had the terrible misfortune of bending over to retrieve an errant spike at the same instant an overly enthusiastic teammate leaped into the air, her arms and legs akimbo. One of her feet whacked him on the side of the head and he hadn't been the same since.

He was tired of taking aspirin, which he wasn't supposed to be taking in the first place because he was planning to undergo surgery for an ulcer. He talked a lot about stress—he was going through a divorce, he had a new girlfriend, he ran the chance of being laid off from his job. Could the stress be contributing to his headaches?

It certainly didn't help, I told him. What I didn't tell him was that his symptoms appeared a little more serious. I began to motion out his neck and spine but didn't get very far. As I applied a tiny bit of pressure to stretch his neck muscles, George cried out in pain. Whoa! What was this?

I stood behind him and began to motion out his spine as he sat on the exam table. Halfway through, he lurched for the wastebasket and began to vomit.

I've had kids throw up on me before, usually after they've eaten an entire family-size bag of Skittles. But I'd never had an adult lose his cookies on me. I helped George with the wastebasket and offered him some Kleenex tissues to wipe his face. He was too sick to even be embarrassed. He didn't care.

My mind raced back to first year anatomy lab at Northwestern. We had mastered the fat and muscles in our cadavers and had moved on to the skull. We were going to study the brain and analyze how the nerves of the spine formed the connection that makes us uniquely human.

Anatomy lab isn't for the faint-hearted or weak-stomached. We used saws to cut through the skull. We cut the skull into two hemispheres, exposing firm gelatinous gray matter that could then be lifted out to study.

But I ended up with a cadaver who had a mind of his own—so to speak. Whoever embalmed the body missed the brain. As I lifted off the skull, the entire contents, which looked like melted strawberry ice cream, but, unfortunately, didn't smell like it, came pouring out. Instinctively, I reached out with both palms and caught the majority of it. The rest slipped through my gloved hands and began to ooze to the floor. I pleaded for help from my classmates, but instead of coming to my rescue, they backed away in horror. Hey, what are friends for?

Sometimes I think that while certain classes were designed to stimulate our intellect, they were also designed to desensitize us to the many unexpected—and unappetizing—events that would befall us when we finally set up our own practices outside those hallowed halls. For that, I am grateful.

But as George groaned, I turned all my attention to him, and my first thought was that the kick during the volleyball game had cracked his skull, or that he had intracranial hemorrhaging, or both.

I wasn't going to do any adjustments on George. There was something wrong here that needed more testing. I performed several orthopedic tests on him, including the Valsalva test, which helps to indicate disc problems. It came out positive.

I also checked for Kernig's sign for spinal meningitis. It came out negative. George had no fever, and he hadn't been swimming recently. His symptoms intrigued me. But even though they were inconsistent, he was still a very sick man.

"George, you're going straight to the hospital. We're going to get you a CT scan."

Since it was noon anyway, I rushed to the hospital along with George and discussed the case with the emergency room physician. He showed me the CT scan. It looked perfectly normal. I was baffled.

"I'd like to do a lumbar puncture," the doctor said. "I'd like to check for spinal meningitis." But I already checked for Kernig's sign, I thought. It came out negative. I had palpated his skull and felt edema while George waited for the results of the CT scan.

You know what? The emergency room physician was right on the money. George had spinal meningitis. I was shocked. What about the kick in the head during the volleyball game? The problems with stress? The negative orthopedic tests?

I sat with the physician in the doctors' lounge and shared a cup of coffee. "How did you know?" I asked.

His grin reminded me of poker games I used to play with my grandfather. He always won. There's a lot of skill involved in card games. You have to remember which cards have been played and which ones are still out there. And there's a lot of luck involved, too. When the right card ends up in your hand, you have to know it's the right card, even before anything else matches it. I began to feel little goose bumps crawling up the back of my neck.

"We had four cases of spinal meningitis in here last week," he replied. His coffee cup blocked his mouth, so I couldn't tell if he was smiling, but he had an unmistakable twinkle in his eye. I could feel my eyes widen. There hadn't been a single case of meningitis for a year, then all of a sudden, four popped up out of the blue. Getting kicked in the head was just a red herring. All my favorite Agatha Christie novels flashed before me, like the lifetime memories of a man about to die.

How many times would a patient's history mess up my head and deter me from a proper diagnosis? And how many times would the history be true blue, leaving me with nothing to do but jot down a few notes and slap a sticker on a file folder?

I'd lost this card game, but I was glad that somebody had won. If I played enough, I knew I could be as good as my grandfather. Besides, he was a lot older.

CHAPTER 27

"Something between a hindrance and a help."

William Wordsworth

It began to get so busy at the clinic that I found myself staying up half the night finishing the paperwork that should have been done during the day. More than that, we'd just found out that Terry was pregnant, and I couldn't concentrate on my work. I was filled with excess energy, running to and fro like a windup toy, making Clara nervous and wearing myself out. I'd counted the days on the calendar and knew that I'd need someone to help me out on the Big Day. If Terry went into labor in the middle of the day, I couldn't just drop my patients and run; someone had to work on them. And I had really planned on taking a couple of days off when the baby came home.

As far as the patient load and office work was concerned, Clara was working out fine, but she only had two hands. I just had to hire another assistant. And a doctor.

The assistant I had no problem hiring. Our building had just opened a training school and students were always looking for jobs. I interviewed a dozen candidates and decided on a very professional woman named Nancy. She had experience as a private nurse and had run a day-care business from her home, but decided to go back to school for medical transcription. She tended toward stockiness, had a pleasing manner and could type faster than anyone I'd ever known.

The doctor, on the other hand, I was going to have some difficulty with. Did I want a partner or an employee? Did I need him every day? Would he develop his own patient load at the clinic? Could he speak at local civic groups, like Kiwanis, Lions and Rotary?

I ran notices at my college out of state and with the Virginia Chiropractic Association. Within a week, I received a call from a young man who had just graduated from a school in another state and was interested in working at a private clinic. I set up an appointment for the next Tuesday and awaited the meeting anxiously.

We'd been so busy lately that I almost didn't care who I hired, just so he could walk, talk and adjust. Someone who could keep an eye on patients while I ate lunch. Someone who could run therapy on people. Someone to talk to when I got excited about a patient who had cervicothoracic joint dysfunction and who actually understood what the words meant.

I know I should have been more patient. I should have waited a few more weeks, interviewed a half dozen candidates, mulled over the choices. But when Fritz Dillard walked in my front door, I had already decided to hire him. I practically fell over myself just walking across the room to greet him. Never mind his diagnostic skills, his x-ray finesse, his ability to adjust; this man represented the first vacation I was about to have in three years!

Having just finished school, he was understandably reluctant to discuss at great length any detailed or baffling case histories. He preferred to focus in on his hours, how many patients we saw each day, and what the pay scale would involve.

He solved my partner/employee dilemma instantly: he had no desire to become a partner. He was just looking for a job. After all, he'd just graduated from school; he didn't want to appear greedy or cocky. I was relieved.

At about six feet, he was my height and had a shock of black hair that curled into his eyes until he brushed it out with a casual sweep of his hand. He spent a lot of time with his hands in his pockets, and stood with one hip jutting out, relaxed, but tough, like a cowpoke.

His eyes were bright green, sparkling whenever he laughed, and his teeth were huge and perfect. He had an odd laugh, more of a chuckle, and it added to his relaxed nature. He'd slow me down, this Fritz Dillard. He was a good foil for my Type A personality.

I gave him a tour of the clinic, and suddenly it occurred to me just how small a place I'd been working in. He brushed up against the magazine table in the reception area and knocked several magazines onto the floor. He apologized profusely, picking them all up, catching them as they slid from his grasp, and plopping them back onto the table in a haphazard fashion. As we walked down the hall, his shoulder nudged an inexpensive fine-art print I'd picked up at one of the museums in D.C. and sent it sliding sideways on its wire backing. It hung diagonally, its bucolic scene reflecting the world from a cock-eyed point of view.

By the time Fritz got to my office, he'd knocked over a plant and spilled the cup of coffee I'd given him.

He's nervous, I thought. That's a good sign; he's humble and knows his limits. But still, it bothered me about the clinic being so cramped. We'd just have to move to larger quarters as soon as my bank account would allow it.

But I had one more piece of business before I could conclude our meeting. "I have a rib out of place and a subluxation at T4," I said. "How about adjusting me?"

He shrugged his shoulders noncommittally and said, "Sure."

We made our way into the nearest treatment room and I lay face-down on the adjusting table. He palpated the area with an expert touch, applying just the right amount of pressure in all the right spots. The "crack" that came with the adjustment was especially pleasing because I hadn't been adjusted in months. I could see his shoes through the space in the face cushions. He was wearing brown leather boat shoes with white soles. One of the laces had come untied and hung lazily over the edge of the shoe. I wondered where he'd been before he'd shown up for the interview.

He'd work out just fine, I thought, excited about the relief I would experience when he began to see patients. "When can you start?" I asked, standing up and adjusting my tie. It was then I noticed that Fritz wasn't wearing a tie—just an open-neck shirt and cardigan. His attire was in direct contrast to my own. I was always buttoned to the top, always wore a tie, which I knotted as tightly as I could, and chose conservative wingtips for my feet—the same kind my father wore long before I was ever born.

"Now," he replied.

"How about Monday?" I suggested. That would give him the remainder of this week to finish up any odds and ends in his personal life. He agreed.

"Why don't you meet me for dinner tomorrow night? I'd like you to meet my wife," I offered.

"Sure," he said, and we arranged to dine at a local Chinese restaurant known as much for its sizzling War Bar as much as its breathtaking stained glass collection.

By the time I sat down to dinner that night, I was so exhausted that my only thought was to crawl into bed. With an effort, I barely managed to sit up straight and carry on an intelligent conversation with Fritz. I shoved food in my mouth without the slightest interest in what it was and sipped tea in a vain attempt to stay awake. Every now and then, Terry would come to my rescue and finish a sentence for me. I'm afraid that I was a total deadbeat when it came to impressing Fritz.

I needn't have bothered. He spent an inordinate amount of time staring at the group of young women seated at the booth next to us. The four of them had been giggling and gossiping for at least an hour, and their noise level rose in direct proportion to the receding level of fluid in their cocktail glasses. "Would you like to stop by the house for some coffee and dessert?" I asked, as Fritz smiled unabashedly at one of the women.

"Fritz?"

"Uh, well, no thank you. I, um, made other plans." The woman he'd been ogling winked, and suddenly it occurred to me that to Fritz I was a definite dud. Who was I to think that this guy, right out of school, would be interested in spending the evening with a couple of duds nearing forty who didn't drink, one of whom was pregnant? I felt old. Months of exhaustion had taken their toll on me. I glanced over at the table next to us, and not a single one of those women held the least bit of interest for me. They were probably good looking by anyone's standards, but it had been so long, I'd be hard pressed to rate them on a scale of 1 to 10.

As we rose from the table, Fritz twisted awkwardly, knocking a cup of tea to the floor, spilling it on his trousers. The brunette he'd been smiling at leaped up and began to blot the spill with her napkin, then stood back stiffly, suddenly realizing how forward she'd been. Everyone broke into laughter, but I could see that this was the opening Fritz had been hoping for.

I glanced at Terry, looking as exhausted as I, but with better reason, and put my arm around her. I couldn't wait to get Fritz to work and spend my evenings sprawled on the couch with the evening paper, while Terry painted in her studio. I lived for the future. The present was on autopilot.

Monday dawned bright and clear, and Fritz showed up at 8 A.M. sharp. We dispensed with the paperwork immediately and set about preparing for patients. "I'll bring you into all the treatment rooms with me today and introduce you to everyone," I told him. You can watch how I do exams, and just kind of sit in. Then tomorrow, you can do a few exams and I'll sit in with you. We'll just take it one day at a time."

There was no doubt in my mind that we'd be set for my vacation by Friday. What a relief! I began to wonder how patients would react to Fritz and was really looking forward to the encounters. Studies show that whenever you hire a new doctor, 30 percent of the patients will prefer him, 30 percent will prefer their original doctor, and 40 percent don't care who works on them. I'd be interested to see how Fritz fit into the statistics.

Our first patient that day was Connie, a social worker who had neck and lower back problems. Since she'd been in before, I did a brief follow-up exam just on her neck and lower back, and immediately put her on therapy. I could see that she was going to get along with Fritz just fine. They were very relaxed with one another—all smiles and friendly nods. Connie giggled a few times and looked down at her feet when she talked to Fritz and, when she looked back at him, blushed. Funny, she never reacted to me that way. Before I'd had time to ponder the idea, another patient came in. I told Connie that we'd be back to take off the therapy in a few minutes and then give her an adjustment.

The next patient was an older woman who'd had a couple vertebrae surgically fused together and was in a lot of pain. Mrs. Bradley's body was filled with arthritis and, on top of it, her cholesterol and triglyceride levels were totally unacceptable. I had put her on an exercise program that included water aerobics and walking and helped her change her diet.

Mrs. Bradley treated Fritz like a kid. I could see that she was trying her best to make him feel welcome, but her manner was condescending. She couldn't help it; after all, she was eighty-two, and Fritz was only twenty-six.

I put Mrs. Bradley on therapy and told her that I'd be back to adjust her. I adjusted only her upper back and neck, since her lower spine was fused. It was especially important to keep all the joints moving. She was already in enough pain and certainly couldn't afford to have her joints freeze up.

We returned to Connie, and I had Fritz remove the electrical stim and cold pack. He palpated the back of Connie's neck very naturally, and I felt good about his easy manner. I adjusted Connie and told her I'd see her in a few days. As I walked down the hall to the next patient, I began to chat with Fritz about the next patient. It wasn't more than two seconds before I realized that I was talking to myself.

I turned around to look, and there was Fritz, walking Connie out to the reception area, helping her with her coat. They looked like a couple on their way out to a nice restaurant. I felt vaguely uneasy.

Fritz soon joined me, and I introduced him to Martin Joseph, an insurance representative. Martin had sprained his shoulder and pulled a muscle playing softball over the weekend. It was simple to diagnose the problem and come up with a treatment plan. My treatment included a lecture on warm-ups before a game. As I talked to Martin about stretching, Fritz walked over to the wall and studied the anatomy posters I'd hung there. He wasn't paying any attention to us at all.

"Dr. Dillard," I said, "why don't you show Martin a few stretches that he can do before his softball games?"

Fritz was visibly startled, but he recovered instantly and walked around the treatment table to stand before Fritz. "Be sure to stretch before your next game, Martin," he said, patting him on the shoulder. I groaned. Martin didn't notice. I could see that Martin was sliding into the one-third "I couldn't care less" statistic.

It occurred to me then that those statistics could apply to doctors as well. Who was to say that Fritz couldn't care less about a third of his patients, or that he'd learn to hate a third? Connie, on the other hand, fit into the favorite third. I began to worry. Was that unethical? Or just human? I mean, how on earth could anyone possibly adore every single one of his patients?

If my hypothesis was true, then I had three alternatives: 1) Get rid of Fritz; 2) Take on all the patients that Fritz wasn't interested in; 3) Teach Fritz my philosophy, which is to try to find something I like about every patient. I met a ninety-year-old retired teacher whose students, now highly successful professionals, all adored her. She was the best teacher they'd ever had. The city had even named a school for her. Her secret? She loved them all, each and every one of them. "I kept a journal," she told me once, "and I found an old entry that detailed the problems I was having with one of my students. He was disruptive, angry, always dirty from head to toe. I finally found something to like about him, but I really had to work at it. Children sense that, you know. Everyone has something good about him; it's your job to bring that out. A good teacher just has to learn to look a little deeper. It's a challenge."

I knew that patients could sense that I was preoccupied or angry simply by my touch; a tenseness in the wrist, or unneccesarily rough palpation. I could teach that to Fritz.

As we left that treatment room and moved on to various patients throughout the day, I could see that, indeed, Fritz was drawn to certain patients more than others. He was young, I thought. This is his first job in a clinic outside of school. I decided to cut him some slack.

By the end of the week, Fritz had invited Clara and Nancy to lunch twice before I'd ever had a chance to arrange it myself. A couple of patients had already expressed an interest in being treated only by him. I hadn't expected that to happen so fast. The female patients in particular were drawn to him. He certainly wasn't shy around women. They were drawn to him, some because he seemed like a son, some because he acted like a brother, and some because he apparently had some sort of sex appeal. I decided to consult with Terry on the subject.

"Sex appeal? Are you kidding?" she laughed. "Why didn't you just hire Christopher Reeve or Michael Douglas? The women fall all over him—even the older ones. He seems so helpless—he's the type you want to pick up after, brush lint off his shoulder, listen to his problems. And those eyes!"

"Then why did one of my older patients condescend so much to him?" I asked. "She acted like she was just tolerating him."

"Well, he is a doctor, after all. She's obviously the no-nonsense type who wants a diagnosis and that's the end of it. She's probably been through eighty surgeries and the last thing on her mind is flirting with a doctor forty years younger than she is."

"She's had a couple vertebrae fused," I said. "You're right. That makes sense."

"Does that bother you?" Terry asked. "I mean, that Fritz is the way he is?"

"No. Why should it bother me. As long as he's a good doctor. . ."

I could see she was trying not to grin. She was teasing me. "I don't feel threatened," I said. "That's not professional."

"What's not professional—feeling threatened because he's so obviously sexy, or threatened because you consider his manner detrimental to your practice?"

"Never mind," I said. My mind was already on other things. Like taking a day off. Just a day. I'd stretch it to a week when Fritz was ready. But a day would be fine for starters. Fritz could handle one day. Sure. No problem. I'd just sleep late and let Fritz handle everything. I'd call in sometime in the afternoon just to see how things were going, and I wouldn't worry about a thing. He could even handle one or two emergencies or walk-ins. He could definitely handle adjustments and therapies. He could even handle the x-rays. And he'd certainly picked up on office procedures. Yeah, he could handle one day. He could do it all. Without me. Maybe I wouldn't even have to call in. Maybe no one would even miss me. No one would even know I was out of the office. They'd just be wanting Fritz. Fritz and his gentle, suave manner, his bedroom eyes, his slightly mussed hair. . .He'd redecorate the office where I'd placed him, of course. Hang up all his own diplomas and family photos and posters and fill the drawers with his own reading material and a few special snacks. I'd probably not even recognize the place when I walked in.

The kitchen phone rang, jarring me from my stream-of-consciousness. "Hello?" It was Connie, the social worker. She'd been rear-ended in her pickup truck and wanted to see me right away, tonight, at the clinic. The hospital had x-rayed her and found nothing broken, so the staff had sent her home. She was in a great deal of pain and didn't want to stay up all night in agony. "Dr. Dillard is a real sweetie," she added before hanging up, "but I really want you to work on me. This is serious. I just know you're the only one who can help me."

As I hung up the phone, a sudden feeling of elation swept over me, a surge of pride and conviction and self-satisfaction. She needed me. What do you know!

CHAPTER 28

"It's been a hard day's night."

The Beatles, song title

Some patients are such agreeable sorts that you really look forward to their visits. They tell jokes and interesting stories. Some bring homemade cookies. Some bring small children who sit in the reception area and entertain themselves by drawing colorful, playfully distorted portraits of the doctors. The assistants delight in taping the drawings to the walls and doors. Some patients seem to get better the moment they walk in the door. And some patients are nice to look at—bodybuilders, aerobics instructors, toddlers with a rainbow of ribbons in their hair.

And then there are the difficult patients. Those who, no matter how often you talk with them, sympathize with them, call them at home, and give them advice, still fail to progress. It's not that their problems are that difficult to treat; it's that, for some reason, they just don't want to get better. They find that they get attention when they're in pain, and they derive sympathy from friends, family and office staff. Or they have so much anger bottled up inside that they are simply unapproachable. Sumi was just such a patient.

Sumi was a petite Chinese woman, born in Hong Kong, who showed up at my office after she'd hurt herself at work. Her back was in such bad shape that she couldn't even stand up straight. I x-rayed her and found dozens of problems. Sumi was in a great deal of pain.

After completing Sumi's first treatment, I sat her down and explained exactly what sort of things she could and could not do in her condition. No heavy lifting. No strenuous exercise. She nodded agreement and said she understood perfectly.

The next day, Sumi came back into the office and I was surprised to hear that she had chewed out Clara at the front desk. Sumi's back hurt and she couldn't do a thing! She couldn't lift heavy objects. She couldn't do any strenuous activities.

I brought Sumi into my office and explained, once again, what it was she could and could not do. As a precaution, I had Sumi repeat the instructions back to me. Thus assured, Sumi was sent on her way.

The next time Sumi had an office visit, I was out of the office and Dr. Dillard treated her. She was his first solo act, and he did his best to accommodate her needs. Sumi told him that her neck and her back hurt and she wanted only certain adjustments. He complied. For such a petite little thing, she sure was bossy. Asking a patient to share responsibility for her care is not the same thing as letting her take over. She has no way of diagnosing herself except to tell the doctor where the pain is. Dr. Dillard became merely a piece of technical equipment that Sumi used to her discretion.

Sumi's next three visits were also with Dr. Dillard. Each time she was scheduled to come in, Fritz cringed when he saw her name in the schedule book. She was a difficult person to deal with, that was for sure. He was getting awfully tired of her complaining and bossing. And she never did any of her exercises and seemed to deliberately undertake activities that would make her condition worse.

During Sumi's next visit, she decided to find Dr. Dillard to speed up her appointment, and wandered from the reception area. She barged into a treatment room and stumbled upon a chubby businessman who, sans shirt and tie, was sitting on an exam table reading a magazine. His gasp and startled face were enough to send her on her way. She chose another treatment room, and found Dr. Dillard treating a middle aged woman. Luckily, the patient was lying face down and didn't see the door open. As discreetly as possible, Dr. Dillard told Sumi to return to the reception area and he pushed the door shut with his foot.

The next time Sumi came by, she stood at the front desk and chewed out Clara again. She wasn't getting any better, she complained. Loudly, she protested that the staff and doctors were simply trying to get her money—that they were taking advantage of her because she was Chinese.

I could hear her all the way down the hall, and my head began to pound. Rather than put her in a treatment room, I brought her into my office.

I instantly addressed the issue of prejudice. I told Sumi that discriminating against Chinese or anyone else was strictly forbidden in my clinic. I explained that hers was a worker's compensation case and the fees paid were the same across the board for her type of injury. Even if I were prejudiced, I could not possibly change the fee.

I told her, in no uncertain terms, that she was welcome to remain my patient as long as she didn't bad-mouth my staff, and that she should address any complaints or questions to me in private. An appointment was scheduled for the next day. Sumi would be treated only by me from now on. Despite my stern manner, she seemed relieved and said she understood.

As if she had absolutely no short-term memory, the next day Sumi sauntered up to the front desk and, at the top of her lungs, screeched about what a horrible clinic this was and how everyone was discriminating against her because she was Chinese. She was one angry woman. The whole world was against her, and it all stemmed from this office.

Patients in the reception area ruffled magazine pages nervously and glanced over their shoulders. There was nowhere for them to run.

I did not treat Sumi that day. I brought her straight into my office and sat her down like a child. Then I handed her the phone book.

"This is so you can look up another chiropractor," I said. "I'd choose one for you, but I don't want any other doctor to blame me when he finds out I referred you to him."

Sumi looked confused.

When patients choose a chiropractor as their "port of entry" to the health care system, he is their primary-care physician and must maintain an open line of communication at all times. A doctor who goes on vacation and who fails to inform his staff and patients may be sued for abandonment. One exception is teaching hospitals, where a waiver is signed by patients who are then sometimes shuffled about between several physicians. I could not cut off Sumi's care without ensuring that she had another doctor to go to. I was very angry, but I wasn't about to let rational behavior escape me.

"You are no longer my patient or Dr. Dillard's patient," I said. "You will no longer be treated in this clinic. You're disruptive, you wander into other patients' treatment rooms, you ignore our advice, and I cannot tolerate your abuse of my staff. Do not come back. Choose another doctor from the phone book."

"All you want is the money from my workman's comp," shouted Sumi, her dark eyes flashing.

"If that's true," I countered, "then why am I refusing to treat you? I certainly can't make money off of someone I am not treating."

Sumi finally got the message and burst into tears. I gave her a tissue and escorted her out the door. It was a great relief to everyone there. Except for Sumi, who was forced, by her own behavior, to find somewhere else to vent her anger and frustration.

Every now and then I think of Sumi and wonder if she's still in pain, if she is still angry with herself and the world. I wonder how many Sumis are out there.

CHAPTER 29

"One should never know too precisely whom one has married."

Nietzsche

When I was growing up, I believed that the perfect doctor's wife was calm, patient to a fault, caring, nurturing, insightful, and always there to listen, to cook, clean and offer a badly needed hug.

The perfect doctor's wife would be pretty, but not gorgeous. She would always say the right thing at the right time. She would be intelligent enough to ask all the right questions and comprehend even the most intricate diagnoses, but not so brilliant that she took away the doctor's shine in public.

The perfect doctor's wife would be the kind of woman who drew people to her, people in need of a good listener, a shoulder to cry on. She'd entertain colleagues at home with exquisite meals, elaborately prepared, and the house would glow with warmth and cheer and an ambience not to be found elsewhere.

The perfect doctor's wife would bake homemade cookies just like my mother had waiting for us when we burst in the door from school. She would have my dinner waiting for me no matter what time I came home. She would rise with the sun, softly pad to the kitchen, and prepare a cup of aromatic coffee to warm my chilly bones and start my day with a smile.

She would laugh at my jokes. She would tell me she loved me and rub my aching shoulders at the end of the day.

I knew I'd chosen the perfect doctor's wife. With a bachelor of fine arts degree in illustration, she was so talented, her work awed me. I'd spend hours staring over her shoulder as she added light to dark, shading just so, creating three-dimensional figures out of mere pieces of paper.

When we began to settle in to our lives in the South, our new friends did their best to help her feel comfortable in this alien environment.

"I love spinach," she told our friend, Katy, one night. Katy had prepared fried chicken, mashed potatoes, grits, corn pudding and an assortment of Southern vegetables in a dizzying array of choices. We were guests that night, included in her family gathering.

"That's not spinach," Katy said. "They're greens."

"What's the difference?"

Chuckles flittered through the kitchen. "Taste them," offered Katy.

"May I have a roll?" asked Terry.

"You mean a muffin?"

"Whatever. One of those flour things like little bread."

"How about some chitlins?"

Stunned into silence at what she recognized as something that would never touch her Yankee lips, Terry simply shook her head.

"We're going to take you shopping," offered Katy. "We're going to get you some proper clothes—you're a doctor's wife now."

Terry's eyes widened. Then she frowned. "What's wrong with what I'm wearing?" she asked.

Everyone at the table cast a look in Terry's direction. Her shoulder length, permed brown hair was drawn up at the side by a pink flamingo hairpin. Matching flamingo earrings dangled against her neck. She wore a pink turtleneck underneath a baggy cream-colored knit sweater that reached to the tops of her thighs. Skin-tight blue jeans were covered at the ankles with shin-high black boots.

"Nothin's wrong with what you've got on," soothed Katy. "But when you go out, you need to have an image. Doctors' wives should look proper when they're standing at their husbands' sides."

"I have dresses," Terry said.

"Well, you need to get yourself some proper clothes."

Terry wasn't altogether certain about the goals that had been set for her by these new friends. She had a better idea.

"Let's go shopping," she told me one Saturday. "You need some clothes."

"I do?"

"Yes," she replied, tugging at my sleeve and grabbing the car keys. "We're going to buy you some new clothes. You have an image to portray. After all," she grinned, "you're an artist's husband."

I suddenly felt a pang of guilt for not rushing to Terry's rescue at the dinner table that night. She'd hardly said anything, but I could tell that it bothered her. The perfect doctor's wife? Certainly not a Stepford Wife, I chastised myself.

I was game. We drove to the local mall and scoured the racks of men's clothes. Off came the starched white shirt, red tie and navy sport coat. We chose an aqua and white striped shirt and a pencil-thin tie to match. Then we found a pair of black wool pants flecked with aqua threads, like candy confetti on a child's cupcake. The cut was very 1940ish—wide hips, pleated in front, tapering toward the ankles, finished with cuffs.

For the grand finale, we settled on a roughly woven sport coat with elbow patches. I was a new man. Where was the *GQ* photographer? We marched right over to Katy's to show off my new ensemble. "What do you think?" I asked, impatiently.

"Wow," said Katy. "Are you going out?"

"No, this is to wear to work." She frowned, confused and somewhat disapproving.

"I have to dress like this. I'm an artist's husband."

Katy shot Terry a surprised and somewhat wounded look. She quickly recovered and laughed the whole thing off. But we'd made our point.

Even so, something pulled at me. Katy was right. Terry didn't really fit in. In some ways, I relished her independence. In others, I wished she'd fade into the background. It wasn't that she was abrasive, it was that she was so, so—so unlike the perfect doctor's wife! The image haunted me months later, when my pager went off near midnight. The shrill beep-beep-beep sliced through the air and awoke us from a sound sleep.

"Whoever it is had better be very, very sick and in a whole lot of pain," moaned Terry from her side of the bed. "If he's not, I'll make sure he is when I'm through with him."

"I have to go to the office," I said.

"*What?!!* It's the middle of the night! Send whoever it is to the emergency room! Why do you need a beeper, anyway? You're the only chiropractor within a thousand-mile radius who has one. What did Whoever-It-Is do, anyway?"

"He was at a party and he lifted a keg and threw out his back," I said.

"*Ha!*" she cried. "He deserved it!"

I sighed and went out the door, wondering if the perfect doctor's wife really existed.

A month later, I dragged myself in the door after a grueling fifteen-hour day. Lingering childhood memories prompted anticipation of a warm meal and bustling household activities. I was promptly jerked from my introspection by Terry's voice. "Where have you been? It's 11:00! I thought you were dead! You certainly couldn't have had patients this late! Why didn't you call?"

"I cured two migraine headaches, sixteen lumbar injuries, diagnosed three cases of thoracic outlet syndrome, sent a case of intracranial hemorrhaging to the emergency room, cured two cases of carpal tunnel syndrome, put a dislocated shoulder back into joint, diagnosed and referred out a case of cancer that the patient thought was a pulled muscle, referred one patient to Overeaters Anonymous, one to Smokestoppers and another to Gamblers Anonymous. Oh, and I referred an axe murderer to a psychiatrist. There was a little paperwork in between and an interview with a local news station, too. Just a normal day at the office. What did you do all day?" I sucked in my breath and waited for a response.

Silence.

"I'm hungry," I said. "Where's dinner?"

"Where *was* dinner," Terry corrected me. "After waiting for you to show up all night, I fed it to the dogs." Sprawled across the kitchen linoleum, they licked their lips, as if understanding her comment, and banged their tails against the hard floor to show their pleasure.

My heart sank. How could she look so vindictive and menacing, not to mention smug, with all those freckles across her nose? Didn't she know I was Super Chiro, born on planet Chiron, sent to Planet Earth to save Earthlings from spinal nerve interference? I'd show her. I'd jump right back into my Chiromobile and zoom right out of town.

"I've worked hard all day and I don't expect to come home and be treated like this," I said.

"I didn't say you hadn't worked hard," came the reply. "All I asked for was a phone call. Why don't you keep a little alarm clock handy at your desk and set it for about 7:00 so you'll know to call me if you'll be late?"

I thought it was a dumb idea and told her so. Some people are born with missing fingers. Some are born with missing parts to their spines. Some are missing chambers to their hearts. Some are born without sight or hearing. Doctors' wives are born without any sense of humor. I went to bed.

The week didn't improve. If it wasn't personal injury cases, it was taxes, and if it wasn't taxes, it was emergencies. If it wasn't emergencies, it was payroll. I was running myself ragged. I decided to go home early for a change.

But when I drove up in the driveway, Terry's car wasn't there. No lights were on in the house. I sat down with a Coke and read the paper. Still no Terry. Being the gourmand that I was, I opened a can of tuna fish and mixed it with some vegetables, eating from the can as I finished the paper. Still no Terry.

I'd been in bed, asleep, for over two hours when I heard her footsteps and the sound of a hanger scraping the dowel in the closet. "Where were you?" I asked from underneath a pillow. "I've been worrying about you all night."

"I can see how worried you are," she chided, "because it kept you awake, sitting at the window, watching for me. I went out to eat with a couple of your cousins and then went to a movie."

"Why didn't you call?"

"What for? You're never here anyway."

"I was tonight. I waited for you all night."

"Oh. Now you know how it feels."

"So do two wrongs make a right?" I asked, indignant.

"No, but they sure prove a point," she replied.

See what I mean? No sense of humor.

The next Saturday night, my pager beeped insistently in the darkness. The alarm clock read 12:15 A.M. "Oh, Gawd," groaned Terry. "Another keg injury." She was having more and more difficulty sleeping now that she was getting so big with the baby, and having the phone wake her just after she'd dozed off didn't contribute to her maternal instincts. It didn't contribute to her sense of humor, either. Maybe that was it—the pregnancy. The pregnancy destroyed her sense of humor! I'd made an incredibly astute medical discovery! What a breakthrough! What a contribution to science!

But it would have to wait. My beeper was beeping. I retrieved the message. It was a false alarm, and a stupid one. One of my patients was drunk at a party and decided it would be fun to leave an outrageous message on my answering machine.

I told Terry as I climbed back into bed. In my somnambulistic daze, I inadvertently let slip the patient's name. "Why would he do such a thing?" she gasped. "Doesn't he know how much noise it makes?"

"I don't think so," I said. "I think he thinks it just leaves a message on the answering machine at work and doesn't know that I carry my beeper with me."

"In the bedroom, no less," Terry snarled.

That next week, we were stretching our legs during intermission in the musical *Annie* when who should be seated behind us but Jason, the prank caller. Although he and my wife had met before, I introduced them again, to maintain the formality. "Excuse us while we get a drink, won't you?" I said, turning and heading for the door. I reached behind me to take Terry's hand and realized that she wasn't there. Separated by the growing throng of people headed for the restrooms, I was helpless to stop her from doing something that I knew was a deeply embedded part of her nature.

As I stared helplessly, she demurely seated herself next to Jason, clasped her hands atop her belly, chatted for a moment, then leaned over, cupped her hand over his ear and whispered something conspiratorially. Jason's hand flew up to his face, and his skin turned crimson. Terry rose, then waved goodbye to him, and, with a wicked smile, headed in my direction. Oh, no, I thought. What did she say to him? I think I'll die. I'll just sneak out during this intermission and not come back.

"What did you say to him?" I asked. "You didn't yell at him for waking us up in the middle of the night, did you?"

"Of course not. You know me better than that. I just asked him if he'd had a good time at the party the other night. He said, 'I sure did. How did you know I was at a party?' I told him I knew because he decided to call and let you know just how much fun he was having. You were right—he had no idea that you carried a pager with you."

"You didn't really have to say anything," I said.

"Yes, I did. Who's to say he wouldn't repeat it again and again until someone told him? Just because you're dedicated to your patients doesn't mean that I am. I need my beauty sleep."

Doctors' wives. Who invented them, anyway?

CHAPTER 30

*"What's in a name? That which we call a rose by any other name
would smell as sweet."*

William Shakespeare, *Romeo and Juliet*

It was Memorial Day and I had been so busy for the past month that
I promised my wife that we would spend the entire day together—just
the two of us. So when my beeper went off, Terry gave me the evil eye.
"It's an emergency," I said, after I'd checked the message. "The
patient's name is Bob and he lives in Hampton. We can stop by there
on the way to the beach. He's in his back yard and he can't move."

That didn't sound too bad. Maybe ten minutes or so, right? We
stopped by the clinic so I could pull Bob's file. I pulled his x-rays,
glanced at them briefly to refresh my memory, and flew out the door.

Terry dropped me off at Bob's door and headed for the local mall.
She was to be back in a half hour. But when she returned, no one was
home, and all she could see was a pillow, blanket, and portable phone
in the back yard. Clearly, someone had been lying there. It looked like
he'd died!

But Bob's kids were at home and said that everyone had gone to the
clinic. Great. So much for a romantic day at the beach.

When Terry got to the clinic, she found the room full of people.
One was the patient's next door neighbor. Her anger began to subside.
If her next door neighbor accompanied her to the doctor's office, it
would have to be pretty severe, she reasoned. Within just a few
minutes, Bob emerged from a treatment room, limping but able to
stand. He and his wife apologized for ruining a vacation day and were
extremely cordial and gracious. Terry was beginning to feel guilty.

After the goodbyes were said, I closed the door and heaved a sigh
of relief. "You're not going to believe what happened," he said. "It was
the wrong Bob."

"The wrong Bob?"

"I know two Bobs. They both live in Hampton. I thought that the Bob who called was a regular patient. But it turned out that it was Bob from my Rotary! I even looked at the wrong x-ray! Boy, was I surprised when I saw who it was lying in the back yard!"

"You didn't tell him, did you?"

"I couldn't help it—I looked down at him and said 'Bob—it's you!'"

It turned out that Bob, the Rotarian, had been overtaken by a sudden bout of industriousness and decided to move the shed in his back yard—all by himself. He soon found out that he was not Hercules, a point that was driven home through the nerves in his spine.

As fate would have it, the two Bobs were destined to meet. I had a New Year's open house at the clinic and they ran into each other over the hors d'oeuvre table. I could feel my face redden as my moment of reckoning had come.

"Bob," I said, "meet Bob. You both live in Hampton and I'll never live *that* one down!" They all had a good laugh, but no one was as relieved as I. I was glad I wasn't a surgeon.

CHAPTER 31

"Oh, what lies there are in kisses!"

Heinrich Heine

Sharon had the hots for me. It sounds like a crude thing to say, but there really isn't any other way to say it. She was not the least bit shy about her intentions.

Sharon was divorced from a man who was doing time in the state penitentiary, and she had an adorable, dark-haired, dark-eyed, olive-skinned three-year-old daughter named Kitty. I just loved that little girl's upturned nose. The mother I could do without. But she did have neck problems, so, keeping in mind the words of advice I'd received from that elderly teacher, I was going to do my best.

Sharon was constantly trying to get my attention. She called often with every complaint in the book. When she finally found herself alone in an exam room with her daughter and me, she'd butt in when I'd tease Kitty or show her any kind of attention. Then, one day, Sharon said her breasts were extremely tender and she thought she'd found a lump. Could I check it out? She hated OB/GYNs and refused to go—even if it meant she was risking her health or even life. What if she had cancer?

Right, I thought. What a come-on. If I did find a lump, my first move would be to refer Sharon to an OB/GYN, so she'd be stuck with an M.D. no matter what. I certainly couldn't perform surgery. But if I did find something, I'd be the only one in a position to persuade her to see a specialist. With my luck, she'd be telling the truth for once and I'd be responsible for neglecting my duties.

I did a breast exam and found nothing to cause alarm. Sharon was perfectly healthy. And very pleased. I was just a tad bit relieved and very angry. I handed her a brochure on breast self-examination and told her to check herself every month.

The next week she complained again. I was too busy to deal with her frustrations—sexual or otherwise—so I did the one thing that all business proprietors have the privilege of doing—I referred her to my associate.

It didn't take her long before she warmed up to Dr. Dillard. Fickle, that woman. I should have known. But poor Fritz.

Not long after, on a Sunday, Sharon called with an emergency. But I never got the call because my pager was on the blink. She called three times and each time left an angrier message than the last. She didn't like being ignored.

Coincidentally, I stopped by the office that Sunday to do some paperwork and glanced at the answering machine. Oops. Lots of messages. All from Sharon.

I returned her calls. She tore into me—screamed and yelled about how she had an emergency and I was ignoring her and she had an excruciating headache. She needed help! I told her to come in. Nope. She would suffer at home. She felt better now that she'd talked with someone. Amazing how she enjoyed Dr. Dillard's company when she was doing fine, but when there was an emergency, only I would do.

I sighed and rolled my eyes heavenward. One minute, it's an emergency and she's *got* to talk to me. The next minute, she's not in enough pain to be seen by the doctor.

The next week, Fritz complained that Sharon was asking him out. Doctors aren't supposed to date their patients, but, on top of it, this woman was a pest, too. How was he supposed to handle the situation? Normally, he enjoyed his role as ladies' man, but with Sharon, it was a different story. Fritz played games; Sharon was serious. He was having a hard time mentally separating Sharon the patient and Sharon the pest. Each time she visited the clinic it became more and more difficult.

Then Sharon started in on Clara. How about dinner and dancing? We can meet some cute guys, have a fun night out.

Clara wasn't the least bit interested. She hated to dance. Hated the cigarette smoke in discos. And didn't really care for Sharon, either. "Maybe next week," said Clara. She didn't want to hurt Sharon's feelings. They continued to chat a bit but I had to shut the door in one of the treatment rooms and couldn't hear the rest of the conversation.

A little while later, I treated Sharon. She told me that she was going out dancing that night with the receptionist but she'd forgotten her phone number. Could I do her a favor and get it for her? I could have sworn that when I'd overhead them talking, Clara said she wasn't interested. But maybe I had heard wrong. And I didn't hear the end of the conversation, either. I shouldn't have been eavesdropping, anyway.

A cardinal rule in this clinic was to never, never, never give out an employee's phone numbers without the employee's permission. But I was tired, busy thinking about the other twenty-five patients I had that day, and fooled by Sharon's apparent sincerity (not to mention relief that she was no longer trying to get me into bed with her), so I mumbled something and went on to the next patient.

The next day, Clara was very cool toward me. She bumped up against me in the hallway, causing me to drop my patient files. I brought her into my office, had coffee and chatted. But Clara wasn't talking about what was bothering her. She seemed nervous and angry at the same time.

So I asked Fritz. No luck there, either. Then I asked Nancy. She said she'd noticed an attitude problem, but had no idea what was going on.

The attitude problem continued for a week. Then Clara called in sick. I was concerned, so I used the front desk Rolodex to look up her phone number. The card was missing. Oh, well, there was another Rolodex in the business office. That one was missing, too. Hmmm. I'd have to look in the personnel file. That card was missing, as well. Uh, oh.

Luckily, I had a personal Rolodex in my office. I called Clara at home and wished her well. I decided that she sounded too sick to deal with questions about the Rolodex, so I passed.

The next week, Clara showed up at work, fully recovered. There was to be a staff meeting that day. The rule in clinic staff meetings was that employees must address all issues immediately. No stewing allowed. In addition, meetings could not be bitch sessions. Anyone with a problem had to also offer a solution.

Willing to give it another try, I asked Nancy if she knew what the problem was. "Yes," she replied. "Someone gave out Clara's home phone number to a patient, and the patient harassed her at home."

Appalled, I gave Nancy a five-minute lecture on what a horrible thing that was and that office policy clearly stated that no one was to do such a thing.

Armed with this information, I approached Clara before the staff meeting. "I heard that someone gave your phone number to a patient," I said. "That is strictly against our policy, and when I find out who did it, there will be hell to pay."

"You did it," she said without blinking.

I blanched. "I did it? When?" Clara explained what day it was and prompted my memory. Indeed, I had. But it wasn't just the fact that any old pesky patient had called a staff member at home. The plot thickened.

When Sharon called Clara, she had no intention of going out dancing. She wanted to pick Clara's brains—because my associate refused to go out with her and said he had another girlfriend. Maybe

Clara could help Sharon figure out who it was. That blonde patient sitting next to the fish tank yesterday? (She didn't know that it was against office policy to date patients.) Another doctor down the street? Maybe he didn't really have a girlfriend—he was just trying to get rid of her.

Through it all, Clara played dumb. She had no idea who it was, she told Sharon. Perhaps she should just give up, because clearly the doctor wasn't interested, and besides, it was against clinic policy.

What she really wanted to do was scream into the phone and shatter the dumb broad's eardrums. "He's *mine,* you numbskull!"—because it was Clara and the good doctor who were having the fling. If only Sharon knew!

It all came out in the staff meeting. My face was red but at least everyone had a good laugh. Clara's name and number are back in all of the Rolodexes, right where they're supposed to be.

Staff meetings will never be the same.

CHAPTER 32

"It's a Mad, Mad, Mad, Mad, Mad, Mad World."

Alfred E. Neuman

When I first interviewed Annette, my office was under construction. We were adding on another section for an additional exam room and x-ray facility. She deftly stepped over the tools and drop cloths, cheerfully brushed powdered sheet rock from her blazer, and followed me into my office to discuss the position.

I was looking for more in an employee this time. I needed someone who knew enough about health care to help patients fill out their consultation forms, answer basic health questions, and distinguish between emergency cases and those folks who just happened to be in a bad mood. I also needed someone who could type letters, answer the phone, run errands, maintain order in the reception area, argue persuasively with stubborn insurance representatives and handle petty cash. I needed a Superman.

Annette seemed perfect for the position. She had a small-town nursing background. She'd raised three boys. She'd taken typing and secretarial courses in college. She was divorced and handled all her own finances. She impressed me with her assertiveness and cheerfulness. She was pretty good-looking, too, except that she wore just a little too much makeup. She had red hair and pale, flawless skin. My gut instinct was that she was a wholesome, gentle lady.

After three interviews, I decided to hire her. She'd never worked for a chiropractor before, but she had worked for an optometrist. I verified her employment there and was lucky enough to catch the head doctor and proprietor.

"I wouldn't hire her again," he warned me, "but my associate would. We have a difference of opinion."

"Why?" I asked.

"When we first started out, there was very little work and Annette handled it well. But then we started to get busy, and she just lost it. She cannot handle a busy clinic."

"Oh, we're pretty small," I reassured him. "I'm sure things will work out fine."

After I hired Annette, the first two or three weeks flew by. She was cheerful and pleasant and loved to visit with the patients in the reception area. Her strong points were her obvious love for children and her compassion for and patience with our elderly patients.

Annette seemed to really care about me, too. She always wished me good morning and good night. She was excruciatingly polite. Every now and then, she'd buy me cookies and make me coffee. But her habit of talking, always talking, with patients and other employees seemed to be slowing her down. Especially now that we were really starting to get busy.

I brought Annette into my office one day and expressed my concerns. "Oh, Nancy was having difficulty with the computer," Annette said, "so I helped her out. She's really very slow, you know."

"I didn't know that, Annette. Thank you for telling me. Why don't you keep an eye on her for me?"

Nancy seemed very competent. I'd never had reason to doubt her skills. But then, I was so busy seeing patients that I hadn't been scrutinizing her, either. Nancy had a motherly aspect to her, which I kind of liked, because it indicated to me that she always had things under control. She seemed especially meticulous.

Annette reported back to me periodically about Nancy's progress. Nancy didn't seem to be getting any better. The problem was that I didn't have the time or interest to manage the computer system, so I couldn't ask Nancy to give me a demonstration. I began peeking into her office and watch her every now and then, and her fingers seemed to fly across the keyboard effortlessly. I wondered why Annette had said that Nancy didn't know the system, but I had to rely on Annette's word.

Weeks went by, and Nancy began to grow hostile. "You're always looking over my shoulder," she complained. "Don't you trust me?"

I had no choice but to back off. I was supposed to be dealing with patients, anyway. I reminded Annette of her supervisory duties once again. "Just what do you tell Nancy when you think she should speed up her work?" I asked Annette. "How do you tell her that she should really know more about the computer?"

"I just tell her," Annette said. She brushed a strand of kinky orange hair from her eyes. Her caked-on gold eye shadow was beginning to wear on me. Twice that week I'd had to tell her to tone down the perfume because it bothered my asthma.

"Does she seem to resent you at all?" I asked. "I mean, does she ever complain that you're looking over her shoulder?"

"Oh, no," Annette said. "Never. We're friends."

"Uh, oh," I thought, "I'll bet that Annette is never telling her anything at all. I'd better have another talk with Nancy."

The next day, I called Nancy into my office. "How is your work going?" I asked.

"It would be fine if you'd just leave me alone," she burst out. "I am an adult, you know. I don't know why you hired me in the first place if you didn't trust me."

"What do you mean? Annette said that you were having trouble with the computer—"

"I know what Annette tells me. And you can just keep your nose out of it. I don't need a babysitter!" She got up and stormed out of my office, slamming the door behind her.

Well, that answered my questions about Annette talking to Nancy; Nancy had verified it herself. Then why the hostility toward me?

The next day, to say that Nancy was cold would be more than an understatement. She didn't even look up when I came into the office. When I buzzed her on the intercom for paperwork, she'd refuse to reply, and then a few minutes later, would appear in my office like a robot and throw the work on my desk. The last straw came when I heard her bad-mouth one of the patients.

"I *said*, you owe us money!" she shouted. "And Dr. Joseph is not going to treat you again until you pay up. Don't give me any of your lousy excuses!"

I flew out of my chair and collided with Nancy in the hallway. "In my office," I said through gritted teeth.

"That's exactly where I was going," she fumed.

"What was that all about?" I said. "You don't treat my patients like that."

"She owed us money and that's all there is to it. You have me working overtime at barely over minimum wage, I've got my hands full, and the more work I do, the more you check up on me and complain about me. I can't stand it any more—I quit!"

That was fine with me, because I was just about to fire her anyway.

When Annette found out, she seemed not the least bit surprised. She didn't seem sad, either. I thought that was odd, since she'd told me that they were friends. Apparently she was more concerned about her date that night.

My next hire would be better qualified, I told myself. I sent out notices to employment agencies and college placement offices.

It was less than a day before names came pouring in. The best qualified was a tall, slender young woman who looked like she could qualify for the cover of *Ebony* Magazine and singlehandedly run the computer system at the Mayo Clinic. Her resume looked good, except that the length of time at any one job averaged three months to a year. Well, she was pretty young—not even twenty-four.

Sheila was an instant hit with the patients. She had an empathetic rapport with those in pain, which was a priceless commodity as far as I was concerned. And she was certainly pleasant to look at with her mahogany skin and luminous brown eyes. But it wasn't long before she started to complain that the workload was getting too hard. "I just can't handle it all," she said. "It never ends."

I just couldn't understand it. There was always one slow day during the week when employees could catch up on the paperwork. When it got really bad, we'd come in on Saturday mornings and have lunch together before heading for home. We were all getting along so well. . .

My lunch hours were often spent chatting with other doctors or business people at the corner restaurant or running errands. Lately, I'd been coming back to a packed office where patients had been waiting twenty minutes before I'd even set foot in the building. I'd even worked straight through a few lunch hours. I couldn't figure it out—everyone knew my schedule by now, didn't they? I felt like a wind-up toy airplane set in motion by a maniacal air traffic controller. Dr. Dillard's work didn't seem to be helping, either.

Annette said that Sheila had messed up the schedule. But the handwriting in the schedule book belonged to Annette. I confronted her. "Oh, Sheila took the call and couldn't find a pencil, so I did her a favor and wrote it in for her," Annette said.

"What about the other names?" I asked.

Annette frowned and looked at the book. "That isn't my handwriting; that's Sheila's."

"Sheila, whose handwriting is this?" I asked.

Sheila walked over and looked. "Why, it's Annette's," she replied. The two women stared at one another.

"Sheila, here's a blank piece of paper. Write down the name Angie J. please. Angie's name was the first one in the appointment book. Sheila complied.

I handed another blank sheet of paper to Annette. "Write down Angie J."

She wrote it down. I held the two pieces of paper side by side. The handwriting in the appointment book matched Annette's perfectly. Her already-pale complexion blanched. The effect was less than becoming.

"Don't ever do that again," I said.

Two weeks later, after taking care of three patients in a row who were in incredible pain, Sheila came into my office, sat down on the couch, and burst into tears. "I can't stand it anymore," she wailed. "My divorce is taking up all my free time, and this office is driving me crazy. All I see are people in pain and people who owe money and every time I look over my shoulder, you're there, watching for my littlest mistake."

I had no idea that Sheila was going through a divorce. That explained a lot about her being on edge lately. Even so, I wondered about the outburst, and sought to contain her fears.

"I think your work is fine, Sheila. I don't know where you get the idea I'm watching over you. I'm with patients all day. If I come into the office to get a patient file, it has nothing to do with you. When was the last time I told you that you weren't doing a good job?"

She didn't answer. I handed her a Kleenex tissue and she sniffled into it while staring at her feet. We both stood up.

I patted her on the shoulder. "Why don't you just take off early today and get some rest. Sometimes things just seem like they add up, but it will be better tomorrow."

She nodded and headed for home. The next day, I was detained downtown during a seminar and had to call the office to have the staff reschedule patients. Some of the later patients could wait forty-five minutes or so, but some just had to be canceled. There was just no way I could get back in time.

I couldn't get Sheila off my mind. I couldn't figure out why she was so flustered all the time when I was the one having an ulcer. How would she feel if she were responsible for a whole roomful of patients in pain and had to take the blame for not taking care of them? All she had to do was pass the buck to me. She was simply a messenger—it wasn't her responsibility.

I rushed into the office around 2 P.M. and instantly began to see patients. Clara was working away at the computer. Annette was orchestrating the reception area and tending to the phones. It wasn't more than fifteen minutes before I wondered aloud where Sheila was.

"She went home early," said Annette. "I, um, think she quit."

Oh, great, I thought. What perfect timing.

The day flew by, and soon it was dark. It was time for Annette to leave as well. Clara was still typing away. She waited to hear the click of the latch as Annette left. "May I have a moment with you, Dr. Joseph?"

"Of course, Clara," I said.

"It was crazy in here today. Everyone was very stressed out. We just didn't know what to do. I wish that if you weren't going to show up for work, you'd tell us."

"I did tell you. I called early this morning and talked to Annette, and then I called back around noon to check on how things were going."

"You did? Annette told us that you called at 1 o'clock."

"No. I know I called because I was in between meetings and I know exactly what time each one ended and began."

"Well, patients in the waiting room were getting angry."

"That's your job to take care of. If it looks like I'm going to be delayed, you take things into your own hands and reschedule. There's no excuse for angry patients. Every single one should be approached and talked to. Just because you're expertise lies in insurance billing and Sheila's forte is the front desk doesn't mean that if one person is out of the office, all hell breaks loose. I trained you all to be able to cover for one another."

"Well, the stress really got to Sheila. And then your wife showed up. We thought she had a message from you, but it turned out she was just dropping something off. Sheila talked with her in your office and came out crying. She said your wife told her to quit."

My eyes widened. What business did my wife have telling my employees what to do? I'd certainly tell her a thing or two. That such a thing would be totally out of character for Terry never occurred to me; I wasn't exactly running on all four cylinders myself at that point.

"Sheila was very distraught," Clara said. "I think she may have provoked your wife. I'm not sure. All I know is that we all had a really bad day."

"Thank you, Clara. I'll be here all day tomorrow, so don't worry about a repeat episode. You shouldn't be here so late. Why don't you go home?"

She looked relieved. I watched her car pull out of the parking lot and wondered what I was going to say to my wife. The office was a mess. I rehearsed a dialogue with my wife as I tidied up. The appointment book was in total disarray—so many names crossed out—and they were in ink, too—they were supposed to be written in pencil. I wondered when the patients had rescheduled and flipped ahead to the next day. Only one patient rescheduled there. Only one for the day after that. None for the week following. What was going on? There were fifteen patients waiting this morning!

I decided to sit down and call the patients myself. If it had been that hectic, it would be more reassuring to hear from me directly.

The first patient answered the phone himself and immediately recognized my voice. "Sitting in your office for an hour and a half in pain isn't my idea of a good time," he croaked. "What gives?"

"I'm terribly sorry for any inconvenience, Mr. Shilling," I replied. He was a construction worker with huge biceps, a big belly, and a short fuse. "I was checking to see if Annette had rescheduled you."

"All she did was gossip with the girls in the back. How do I know it won't happen again?"

"Things come up, Mr. Shilling. I was delayed at a meeting. It sounds like you're really in pain. I'd like to take care of that. I can help. Would tomorrow at 10 A.M. be a good time? It's pretty slow then, and it will give me extra time to look you over."

His attitude softened. "Yeah, that'd be good. See ya then."

I hung up the phone and wondered why Annette was ignoring patients in the waiting room. I needed to pay more attention to Annette. I punched in the next set of numbers. "Hello, Mrs. Pendleton? This is Dr. Joseph. I'm sorry about making you wait today. Could you come in tomorrow around 11 A.M.?"

"I was wondering why that receptionist of yours didn't reschedule me," she said, "but she was more interested in gossiping with the girls in the back. Yes, tomorrow at 11 would be fine."

The other ten calls were nearly identical. What the hell had happened in my office while I was gone? It must have been a zoo. I shuddered.

When I looked at my watch, it was half past 9 o'clock and I realized I hadn't had anything to eat all day. I headed for home, stopping for a hot hoagie on the way.

Halfway through the front door, it occurred to me that I hadn't come up with anything to say to my wife about her conversation with Sheila. I'd really wanted to script myself, to avoid a confrontation. But it was too late. I could see Terry in the kitchen, nursing a cup of tea and poring over a pile of magazines, ripping out coupons.

"You really can pick 'em," she smirked, glancing at me sideways. "Did Sheila have permission to leave the nut house before you hired her or did she escape?"

"What happened?" (Keep her on the defensive, I thought; I'll have more control over the conversation if I field her questions with questions.)

"I stopped by your office today to drop off a folder full of insurance forms for you to sign, and all three of your employees cornered me in your office. Clara was white as a sheet and tightlipped, Annette was babbling incoherently, and Sheila was near hysterics. They all wanted to know where you were and what they were supposed to do with all the patients up in front."

"What did you tell them?"

"I shrugged my shoulders and said, 'I don't know. I don't work here.'"

It was my turn to smirk. Her innocent, squeaky voice and little shrug of the shoulders always made me want to hug her. I felt suddenly guilty for my initial anger at the office. How could I have allowed the staff to make me doubt my wife? Was I being manipulated? Naw, it was just a stressful situation. It could have happened to anyone.

"Then what?" I asked.

"I said, 'If you're so concerned about all the patients in front, why are you all back here with me? Why aren't you rescheduling them?' Clara immediately excused herself and got to work. Annette babbled a little more and left. Sheila stayed in your office with me and shut the door. She cornered me."

"Clara said you told her to quit."

"What?! She told me she was going to quit and that she didn't know what to do. I told her that she didn't need my permission—I didn't even work there. I suggested that if she felt that strongly about it, she type up a two-week notice for you and discuss it with you tonight. I've never seen anyone so distraught. You'd have thought someone just shot her family or something. She was absolutely hysterical—crying, gasping for air. She was shaking uncontrollably. What did she tell you?"

"She wasn't there. She left me a scribbled note that said she was quitting right then and there, and I never even saw her today."

"Oh. Well, good riddance. You certainly don't need employees like that. I think that Sheila and Annette are the reason why your patients were so upset. Clara appeared to be doing her job. Is Sheila always like that?"

I didn't answer. What was it with my hiring practices that was getting me such duds? Their resumes were great. Their interviewing skills were pleasant and polished. Their first few weeks on the job were perfect, if a bit slow. And then, after a certain point, everything seemed to fall apart. Maybe I should have someone else do my hiring. A recruiting company or something. But they're so expensive. Maybe I could take a course in hiring practices. But where would I find the time? Was it me? Did I drive people too hard? Was there something wrong with my personality?

I had no idea how long I'd been sitting in the kitchen by myself, but suddenly I noticed that all the lights were out and my hoagie was cold.

CHAPTER 33

"The lady doth protest too much, methinks."

William Shakespeare, *Hamlet*

Things calmed down a bit after the Sheila episode. I heard that she'd gotten a secretarial position down the street. After thinking about it, I realized that I should have been forewarned by her resume—the longest she'd stayed at any position was a year, the shortest, three months. She'd stayed with me three months.

I had a staff meeting and went over every possible nook and cranny I could think of with Annette and Clara to ensure that the situation was never repeated. They were pleasant and accommodating and things improved with our patients.

And then Capt. Ely came in. Capt. Ely was a former F-15 pilot who had strained his neck repeatedly during flights. His helmet weighed a ton. And those G-forces were awesome. Every time a pilot takes off, the G-forces are the equivalent to being rear-ended in a car accident and getting whiplash. If Mr. Ely complained too often of neck problems to the doctor on base, he'd be grounded. So he came to me.

Capt. Ely's neck was a mess. He had ligament damage and his natural curve was almost nonexistent. I put him on a program of adjustments, alternating ice and heat, and traction. Since he had also messed up his lower back, I put him on ice and heat for that, too. I put Annette in charge of the ice packs and heating unit. She had done that type of work before and seemed to enjoy it.

Capt. Ely came in at 10 A.M. I adjusted him, chatted a bit, put him on neck traction for seven minutes, then brought Annette in the room to help with the ice packs and heat for Mr. Ely's lower back. I told Annette to keep him in the treatment room for twenty minutes. After removing the ice and heat, she was to book him for another appointment and then send him home.

At 11:30, I noticed that the door to room 5 was still closed. I'd been running from room to room in a rush that morning, and all of a sudden, I realized that I should have been using that room, as well.

I tapped gently, and pushed the door open. There was Capt. Ely, sound asleep, his snores punctuating pauses in the piped-in music. I cleared my throat. His eyelids fluttered. I began to remove the therapies. The heating unit and ice pack were both room temperature and very soggy.

Capt. Ely was barely aware of what room he was in. I'd never seen anyone so sound asleep. He seemed a little embarrassed. I palpated his neck, massaged the muscles a bit. He was certainly more relaxed than when he'd first come in. He ought to be, after sleeping more than an hour!

"I can't believe I fell asleep," he sighed. "Must have needed it! I feel great! You know," he added, "that little Annette is cute. She patted me on the shoulder and chatted about all sorts of things before she left the room." He chuckled. "Told me I didn't have to pay the bill, too." He winked. I blanched.

"I'm glad you feel so much better, Captain. Tell you what—tomorrow, I'll take care of your therapy personally."

As soon as he left the clinic, I called Annette into my office. I had to get her off the phone to do it. It sounded like a personal call—too many endearing terms for a patient.

"You left Capt. Ely in room 5 with ice and heat for over an *hour!*" I shouted. "I told you twenty minutes. What were you *doing?*"

"Oh."

"Oh, what? Answer my question."

"I was up in the front. We were busy this morning."

"No kidding. I treated all those patients you sent back and I didn't forget about *them.* Capt. Ely should have been sent home long ago. What is wrong with you?"

Annette had just recovered from strep throat. She'd caught every cold and bug that existed in the past few months. We were beginning to worry about her. Maybe she wasn't getting enough sleep. But I refused to soften. Forgetting about patients is inexcusable. Annette needed to pay attention.

"You're not doing anything with patients any more except escorting them to treatment rooms," I said. "And why did you tell Capt. Ely that he didn't have to pay his bill? Are you insane?"

She said nothing. "Get back to work," I ordered.

I was livid. I should have known better. I should have hired a therapist just to work on patients and kept the other assistants up front. I'd really had high hopes for Annette. Her resume led me to believe that she'd make a great office manager. Now, it was all she could do to show up for work in the morning.

The next morning, Clara called to say she wouldn't be in—her mother had died suddenly. Her mother had lived in New Mexico and Clara was flying out for the funeral. "I'm really sorry, Clara," I told her. "I hope everything goes all right in New Mexico. Let me know if you need anything."

That left me alone with Annette for at least a week. I had left open forty-five minutes three days in a row to conduct interviews, and the rest of the time I would see patients.

I told Terry about my predicament, and Terry surprised me by offering to help out one day at the office. She said she'd answer the phone and book appointments. Terry had always been careful to keep her career separate from mine and had often voiced concern over being placed in a subordinate position. I had lots of colleagues whose wives worked for them, and it worked out great, but then Terry never was cut out to be the perfect doctor's wife. . .I loved her and was very proud of her. But sometimes, she could be so obstinate. Offering to work the front desk was just what I needed.

She seemed particularly interested in my billing procedures and the thought made me chuckle. I've heard it said that if you want your collections up, ask your spouse. Vested interest and all that.

"Clara's mother died," I told Annette. "She won't be in for a few days. What a shame. Anyway, there will be a lot of work to do while Clara's gone."

"I'll call her," Annette responded.

"Don't you dare," I fairly shouted. "She's in enough emotional pain as it is. Leave her alone." I was surprised at my own self-righteousness, but where Clara was concerned, I bristled with protective indignation. I was also getting indignant about myself—it was my office that Annette was messing up.

But I had to attend to the business end of things. I abruptly changed the subject. "How are our collections?"

"Fine, Dr. Joseph. Right on target." Once a month, we set goals for collections, and it was Annette's responsibility to make sure those goals were met. Collections were our sore spot. It had taken me several months when I first opened up my practice to feel comfortable with the idea of people paying me to do something I loved, but after seeing a couple patients use their insurance Med-Pay to buy new cars rather than pay me for several months of treatments, I wised up. I would be no use to anyone if we couldn't pay the rent and had to return all of our equipment.

"What were our collections last month, Annette?" I pressed.

She busied herself with the appointment book. "I'll look it up for you," she said, keeping her eyes lowered. Her eyelids revealed a new shade of blue. Sure beat that tacky gold, I thought. Then again, maybe it didn't.

Just then, a patient walked in. I moved to a treatment room and got to work. Then two more patients came in. Pretty soon, it was lunchtime. Annette's spot at the front desk was empty and the answering machine was plugged in. I'd catch her later.

Around 4 o'clock, I approached her again. "Annette, may I see the collection printout from last month?"

"Sure," she replied. "Just let me get this phone call."

The phone call turned into two phone calls and another patient walked in. I didn't think of collections again until the next day.

"Annette, please put the collection printout on my desk. I wanted it yesterday."

"Yes, Dr. Joseph."

The printout wasn't there by noon. I was getting aggravated. "Annette, where's the collection printout?"

"Oh, I'm sorry—it's been so busy—"

"Get it for me now."

I stood over her while she flipped on the computer. "Why wasn't the computer on this morning?" I asked. "This is the first time all day you've turned it on?"

"Oh, I just turned it off when I ran to the ladies' room. It saves electricity."

The phone rang. A patient walked in, followed by a water cooler salesman. The printout never showed up.

When Terry's day was over, she seemed greatly relieved. I knew that she'd been bored out of her mind. She wasn't a crowd pleaser, and tended to keep to herself, painting. But she seemed relieved for another reason, too. I couldn't quite place it. No matter. I didn't have the time to waste picking through her introverted emotions.

As the sun started to set and the last patient left, I moved up to the business office in search of Annette and the elusive collection statement. But Annette had already left for the day. I decided to phone Clara to see how she was doing.

"Better, thank you," she said. "It's pretty rough. Annette called today, too. She's having a lot of boyfriend problems, so she needed to talk about that, too."

So, Annette went ahead and called from the office despite my warning. "I thought she called up to see how you were doing. Sounds like she spent more time talking about herself."

Clara laughed good naturedly. I remembered that my wife had mentioned to me that she'd run into one of Annette's boyfriends at a local restaurant. She had instantly labeled him a scum ball and couldn't figure out why someone as sweet as Annette would bother with him. Weeks later, Annette complained to the staff and a couple of patients that he called her at home at all hours, begging to come over to have sex. I vaguely wondered where people found the time to do that sort of thing so often in between all their other activities. That explained why she was losing so much sleep and getting sick so often. But I still couldn't figure out why she flip-flopped from acting so sweet and innocent to being such a sexual barracuda. I was no psychologist, but I could see that something was awry.

"Just how long did you talk?" I probed. "Oh, about forty-five minutes," Clara said. "Annette told me that it was her lunch hour."

I sucked in my breath. Annette had left the building during her lunch hour. That meant she'd spent an additional forty-five minutes on the phone with Clara—long distance! And on top of it, she'd left early two days in a row.

"Do you think you'll be in next week, Clara?" I asked.

"Yes. There isn't really much to do here now. My sisters are taking care of selling the house. Now I know that I really want to stay on the East Coast. There's nothing to bring me back to New Mexico any more."

I could hear the pain in her voice and also felt honored that we were beginning to feel like family to Clara. I was beginning to appreciate Clara more and more. I couldn't wait to get her back.

CHAPTER 34

Crazy Like a Fox

Book title, Sidney Joseph Perelman

I'd found a couple of good prospective employees and scheduled an interview with one at lunchtime. I wanted Clara to meet her. My eyes kept wandering to my left wrist and the minutes ticked toward noon. When the waiting room was empty and there was no sign of Annette, I walked over to the computer. It was cold and lifeless.

Clara walked in. She looked so vulnerable and sad after her ordeal, but her eyes sparkled with intelligence and an honest friendliness that I had somehow missed during her absence.

"Hi, Clara. You look pretty good." It sounded like a dumb thing to say, but it filled the silence. Business was always my forte. "Say, just how much electricity does it save by turning off the computer when you go to the ladies' room or out to lunch?"

"You're not supposed to do that," Clara said, her green eyes widening. "The guy who sold it to us said that it was better to leave it on and just turn it off all night. Why?"

"Annette said just the opposite."

Clara looked at the ground. "I don't want to hurt anybody, Dr. Joseph, but I got to thinking while I was gone, that it's about time somebody said something. Annette hardly knows how to operate the computer. She leaves it off all the time so she doesn't have to think about it. Nancy used to have to help her with the program constantly."

I was astounded. "But Annette told me that Nancy didn't know the program and that she was falling behind in her work because of it. And Annette went through a two-week training program."

"She still didn't have a good grasp of it after two weeks," Clara said. "I know that Nancy was helping Annette because I could see them working right behind me. And," she looked up at me, then looked down again, "I've been helping her, too. To be honest with you, it's hard to get my own work done when I'm trying to do Annette's, too."

I was totally confused. "Clara, could you print out our collections from last month?"

"Sure."

She flipped on the computer, loaded it up with paper, called up the program and printed out the month's listing. The whole thing took less than four minutes. I glowed. This was worth waiting for. I could just see everything now—we could pay off the x-ray equipment six months early, give everyone raises, and buy those nifty patient education brochures I'd had my eye on for the past few weeks.

I scanned the page. I scanned it again. Maybe I'd misread it. My eyes bored into it as I read it slowly, carefully, line by line. Last month's collections had fallen 25 percent. We had only collected 50 percent of our total charges. Our goal was 90 percent. Annette had lied to me!

I counted to ten. "Clara, could you please print out our collections for the past six months? Put everything on my desk, and then I'll go over it with you."

I dreaded what the reports would say. Where had all the time gone? I'd been so busy putting out fires that I hadn't even thought about the rest of the business. Why hadn't my school provided me with business classes? It wouldn't have helped me with Annette, anyway, I rationalized. I was really going to have to take some action. I closed the door to my office and practiced hitting the wastebasket on the other side of the room with crumpled pieces of paper. It wasn't the best way to deal with frustration, but it was better than nothing. If I screamed, Clara would either call the paramedics to save me or the police to shoot me.

As I skimmed the reports, Clara confided in me. "Dr. Joseph, Annette seems like such a nice person. That's why I can't figure out why she bad mouths you so much."

My stomach turned inside out.

"I beg your pardon?"

"She told me that your patients could get well all by themselves. And that you were rich and didn't really need the money, so she'd let patients go without paying."

"Why didn't you tell me?" I gasped.

"I thought you knew. Annette said you'd discussed it together. I thought it was kind of strange."

"No, we didn't discuss it. Does that sound like something I'd do? Why would I come to work every day if my techniques didn't work or if I couldn't diagnose? She's crazy! I help people get out of pain. I help get them well. I help them stay healthy. You know how it works around here. You've seen the patients yourself. Why would they come back if their adjustments weren't working?"

But I was lecturing the wrong person. Don't shoot the messenger, I reminded myself. Clara looked taken aback and somewhat sheepish. She was kneading a Kleenex tissue and little pieces were falling onto her lap.

Suddenly, I remembered that my wife had told me something about Annette, as well. Something that Mandy, the health food rep, had told her. Annette and Mandy spent a lot of time together talking at the front desk, and had even had lunch together. Mandy and my wife knew each other because my wife shopped at her store for our personal needs.

Through Mandy, Terry had learned that Annette was suspicious that I was defrauding a particular insurance company by faking patient visits. I was livid. Not only because Annette had concocted such an outrageous lie, but because my wife seemed to wonder if it were possible. No wonder she'd volunteered to work the front desk that day—she wanted to see for herself how the system worked. How could she doubt me? Of course, I had doubted her only a few days earlier during the Sheila episode. Something about the atmosphere around the office was messing up our relationship. The normal flow of events was skewed. Instead of focusing on patients and treatments, I was spending an inordinate amount of time putting out fires. Annette was pitting us all against one another, and she was sneaking out behind the smoke and mirrors.

I couldn't put the insurance lie out of my mind. I replayed explanations through my mind over and over like a VCR. Even if I were attempting such a thing, the patients would find out because the insurance company always sends a copy of the bill to them. Certainly, they'd call to complain, and Annette would be the first to get their calls. I would never set myself up like that. Besides, I could lose my license!

But that was months ago, and I hadn't heard anything since. And I certainly couldn't approach Annette, because the story had gotten so far down the grapevine that it could have been totally distorted by the time it got to me. I had no proof. Did I? I was just rationalizing. Again. Wasn't I?

"Hello? Hello?"

A woman's voice floated through the hallway. It was Catherine, our new applicant. What time was it, anyway? Clara and I welcomed our prospective employee.

About average height, Catherine had pale white skin and long, jet black hair that she occasionally swept back from her high forehead with a graceful hand. Her black eyes seemed never to blink, and never to miss anything. Her eyelashes were thick and black. Without the makeup I'd been noticing so much on Annette lately, Catherine looked credible and refreshingly businesslike. Her handwriting was not only graceful, it was exceptionally easy to read. She was great at math. She'd worked for a dentist and optometrist. Her only drawback was that she seemed a little too drawn, a little too serious. But when she smiled, she absolutely glowed. It wiped out her drama completely.

Clara approved immediately. They seemed to warm up to each other in a way I'd never seen Annette do. Annette was bubbly, cheerful and playful, but there was something plastic about her. Whatever it was that made Catherine so serious also made her very sincere. Maybe it was her handshake—so firm and honest. And Clara stood up so straight when she talked to her. When people talked to Annette, they slouched and giggled and shuffled their feet. It was almost like everyone was flirting with Annette. I'd never really noticed it before.

I trusted Catherine instantly, but my instincts had been proven wrong before. That's why it felt so good to bounce things off of Clara. I told Catherine that I'd call her and that she should think about what kind of a salary she expected. The meeting was the one bright spot in my day.

After Clara and Catherine left, I rushed to read to last several months of reports before Annette got back from lunch. I don't know why I bothered to rush—Annette was late again. The reports were just as bad as I'd dreaded. I picked up the phone and called a temporary agency, and requested an individual who could work for about a month just doing collections. There was just no way I could let this go any longer.

I heard someone in the reception area. Anticipating Annette, I shoved the reports in my desk and hustled to the front. It was Joe, the dog trainer. He'd hurt his back trying to wrestle with an energetic mastiff. I brought him into a treatment room and examined him. Those lower back muscles were really tight. I did an adjustment and decided to put him on electrical therapy. I hooked him up for seven minutes, and ran up front to see if there were any more patients.

Empty.

I returned to the treatment room and chatted with Joe for the remainder of his treatment. He seemed better, but I warned him to watch his back. "Why don't you tell people that you only obedience train Yorkshire Terriers?" I asked. "It would be better for your back."

Joe shook his head and chuckled. "I can't stand their yapping," he replied. "Give me an old, croaking, powerful bark any day. I want a real dog. Besides, I actually hurt my back more with little dogs because I have to bend down that much more." Annette's ignorance of chiropractic ate away at my insides, and Joe's faith in me, his speedy recovery (one visit!) and his down-to-earth attitude calmed me down. He was a great guy. I was glad he came in.

I walked out with Joe and he asked me to schedule another appointment for him, to make sure he was healing properly and there were no setbacks. (Provided he didn't dance with any more mastiffs!) I marked his name in the book for billing purposes. He'd been gone five minutes when Annette finally showed up, forty-five minutes after she was supposed to. Her makeup was smeared. At first I thought she'd been crying. On closer inspection, I noticed that her lipstick had been wiped off and her necklace was missing. She was fidgeting with her belt. I grew concerned. Was she hurt?

Just as I walked over to her desk, I noticed the single red rose and the note casually tossed on top of the computer. I sighed with relief. And then I got angry.

"Annette, you're late. You can't continue to show up late, take long lunches and leave early. I'd like to see you in my office before you go home."

She started to object, but a patient walked in, and I turned on my heel and left.

Sometime later, Annette disappeared for about fifteen minutes. While she was gone, I treated Lisa, a ballet instructor who had pulled a hamstring. She had improved greatly since her last visit, so she was in and out of the office in a flash. I placed the appropriate mark in the appointment book to indicate what sort of treatment she'd received so that Annette could do the billing.

Soon after, Annette returned with Mandy, our health food store representative. Mandy shot me an angry look and left the office. "Where were you?" I asked her, following her out into the hallway. "In the ladies' room," she said, and walked away. I gave up. I didn't have time to worry about it.

At 5:15, I still had three patients in treatment rooms but decided to run up front to catch Annette. She was on the phone with Joe. She was asking him something about money.

I waved to her and pointed sternly to my watch.

At 5:30, worried that she'd play a disappearing act, I ran up front again. Annette was putting on her coat. "Annette," I said, "I told you that I'd like to see you before you went home."

"But you have patients," she replied.

"You can wait until I've finished. Go sit in my office."

Working on patients when your mind is on other things is extremely difficult. You miss things. You have to perform mundane tasks repeatedly because you can't remember whether you've done them. I was really beginning to dread coming to work every day.

At long last, I locked the front door and met Annette in my office. She was still wearing her coat. She'd repaired her makeup. And prepared a speech.

"I'm really sorry about my long lunch hour, Dr. Joseph. I'm just really sorry."

"That's not what I brought you in here for," I said. She looked bewildered.

I opened my drawer and pulled out the collection reports. "You lied to me. You told me that our collections were right on course. They're not even close. And I asked you repeatedly to get me just one month's report, and you never did. I had to get someone else to get it for me."

"It's been awfully busy, Dr. Joseph. I really have problems juggling everything at once. Your office is too busy to just have one or two staff people."

"Why didn't you tell me before? We have meetings every week. Besides, we're in the process of hiring another person."

"I know."

"But you didn't tell me you were overwhelmed. I need to know so I can do something about it."

"I know."

I frowned. Was this some kind of game she was playing? "I'm getting an outside person to do the collections through this month, to catch up."

"Oh, good." The usurpation of her duties totally escaped her.

"I'm documenting this meeting and putting it in the personnel file." I paused. "Why did you call Joe this afternoon?"

"What do you mean?"

"Joe, the dog trainer. I worked on him during the noon hour. I heard you talking to him about money."

"What do you mean?"

In times of stress, the human mind often tends to muddle and confuse things. But now and then, extreme stress can create a perfect environment for genius. Such an environment was clearly present. At that moment, I had a sudden flash of insight.

"Annette, come up to the front desk with me." I led her to the appointment book and pointed to Joe's name and the billing symbol I had placed beside it.

"You were calling Joe to confirm my treatment today, weren't you? You didn't believe that I really worked on him."

"I never saw him," she replied.

"Of course not. You were late from your lunch hour again. I treated him and signed him up for another treatment and you had no way of knowing whether he was here or not. And what about Lisa? Did you call her, too?"

That was an unnecessary question, because Lisa's Rolodex card was sitting right on top of the appointment book.

"I was here when Lisa supposedly came in," Annette sneered. I'd never seen this side of her before.

"Yes, you were," I said. "But you were gossiping in the ladies' room with Mandy, so how could you have known she was here? You totally missed her."

"You couldn't have treated her that quickly."

"Want to make a bet? You were in the ladies' room for twenty minutes."

"I was in there for five minutes."

"No way."

Annette's face reddened. I could see that she truly believed she hadn't been gone that long. My, how time flies when you're having a good time, I thought.

"Why wouldn't you ask me about this instead of jumping to conclusions and then gossiping to other people?"

"I don't know." Her blue eyes were blank. I believed her. She really didn't know. She just reacted.

She looked down at the ground and said nothing.

"I'll see you tomorrow, Annette." I tried to make it sound like a warning.

After Annette left, I pulled her resume. I replayed the events that led to hiring her. I tried to remember what the other doctor had said. "She can't handle a busy office and doesn't understand technical equipment." I'd been warned. I just hadn't listened. But that didn't explain her attitude, the way she mistrusted me.

Tomorrow. Tomorrow was another day.

CHAPTER 35

"When something good happens it's a miracle and you should wonder what God is saving up for you later."

Marshall Brickman

Amber was a housewife who had injured her neck in a car accident. She was a little on the whiny side but, in general, a pretty good patient. It was her son we had problems with.

At six months old, he was a screamer, a whiner and an absolute complainer. Nothing was ever right for David. He was a cute baby, as babies go. But whenever his mother came in for a treatment, she'd always bring him along. Babysitters were so expensive, after all, and Amber was divorcing her husband and money was tight. Her husband was a patient, too, from the same car accident.

So Annette became the chief cook and bottle washer whenever David came in. I'd treat Amber, listening to her complain about what a louse her soon-to-be-ex-husband, Tom, was, and David would scream his head off in the reception area. We were getting to the point where we were going to have to tell Amber not to bring him anymore. But sometimes Annette would be able to calm him down, and we'd go back to thinking that maybe he wasn't that bad.

That particular day, David was the devil himself. I could hear his wails all the way down the hallway. Then, suddenly, he quieted. I could hear the phone ringing again. And the music running through the intercom system. Had Annette calmed him down?

My wife had slipped in for a moment to have me take a look at her jaw. She'd been visiting friends, and when she bent down to pet their Doberman pinscher, the dog leapt up and sloshed her face with a wet tongue. In the process, he'd smacked up against her jaw and shoved her TMJ out of place.

When I brought her back to a treatment room, she commented on

David. "Who's brat is he?" she asked. "How can you stand all that noise? How does anyone get anything done? Boy, Annette sure had to work at calming him down. She was feeding him a bottle and scheduling patients and answering the phone all at the same time. She sure earned her paycheck this week! Sort of makes up for the fact she's been such an airhead, doesn't it?"

Incredible, how Terry had no difficulty talking with a TMJ out of whack. Sometimes she amazed me.

But she was right. Annette had done a great job. I was impressed. And relieved. She really had things under control. But what was I going to do about her? I certainly couldn't fire her because of her past. Except that her reputation and habits seemed to have a way of catching up with her. Not to mention the fact that she was spreading rumors about me.

I needed to take back my clinic. I couldn't let one good day color my judgment, weaken my resolve. Annette had to go.

CHAPTER 36

"When angry, count four; when very angry, swear."

Mark Twain, *Pudd'nhead Wilson*

Annette was late for work again. She'd called in sick three times last week and twice the week before. This week, at least she was showing up, but she was never on time. I reprimanded her several times, and it did no good. I didn't have to ask her why she was so ill and why she'd been coming in late. I could hear her telling the other employees, my wife, and friends on the phone. Her supposed boyfriend loved the nightlife, and he was wearing her out. Mostly they just stayed home and had sex, but sometimes they'd go out dancing.

Even when they weren't together, he'd call her at home at all hours of the night, she said, and talk and talk. She simply wasn't getting any sleep. She'd tried to put him off by saying she had to go to aerobics, but when she'd get home around 9:30, he'd be waiting at her door and she felt obligated to let him in. This must have been the guy my wife had told me about.

Now, he was calling her at work and disturbing her. I had to ask Annette not to take his calls. She said that was fine with her—he was getting to be a pest anyway.

I couldn't very well fire someone simply because she had a rip-roaring sex life. But the repercussions were hitting the clinic. Her schedule was interfering with my schedule.

Her co-workers and my wife all wondered why she didn't just dump the guy. They'd all seen him around town with a variety of other women. Geez—he probably had a disease or something! What a creep.

But Annette seemed incapable of learning. Finally, he left town, and everyone heaved a sigh of relief.

The next week, a patient told me that Annette had just joined her church and immediately started telling people that she had been approached by the minister. "She's a slut," the patient said. "I don't think you should have her working here."

Such strong language surprised me. I was getting the distinct impression that this was far more than an isolated private vendetta. I was seeing a pattern. In a strange way, it made me feel a little better; at least I wasn't the only one Annette hated enough to start rumors about.

Annette left that church, and was soon seen at a fast-food restaurant with a Christian counselor. This time, it was a buddy of mine, Frank. Oh, no—not him, too! I ached inside. No, maybe they were just chatting and eating fast food. On the surface, it looked innocent enough. Maybe I'd give him a call and warn him. Maybe I should just stay out of it. Maybe I'd ask Terry.

"I don't know who this counselor person is, so I can't help you there, but in general, I think Annette is a nympho. I ran into a dentist friend of yours the other day, by the way," Terry said. "He said that Annette is an airhead and she's screwing up your front desk. He said that it reflects poorly on your business—whoever answers the phone is always a person's first reflection of the business."

"She's not supposed to be answering the phone, anyway. She has other things to do."

"Get rid of her."

"I trained her in. I'm just not giving her enough time."

"It's been almost a year. She's not your daughter. You don't owe her anything. Why do you keep paying her a salary? You should be subtracting the hours she never shows up."

"She's already used up all her sick days and vacation days," I acknowledged. "I don't know what to do. I'll think about it."

It wasn't any picnic having to deal with the mess at the clinic and then having to come home and be lectured by my wife. Even if she was right. I really liked Annette. I found it hard to believe that the things she was doing were really deliberate. She was just overtired, I rationalized. I'd talk with her.

I called Annette into my office and asked if her workload was still too heavy, now that I'd given the collection reports to an outside agency. She said no, everything was fine. I frowned.

"You've got to quit coming in to work late," I chastised her. "I can put you on part time, if that would help." I knew that she was constantly broke, and the thought of a part time job terrified her. Maybe the threat would do the trick. Lord knows, I'd tried everything else.

"Oh, no," she burst out. "Full time is fine. I'll make up the hours on Saturday."

Annette was on salary. She didn't really have to make up the hours, since it was a given that some days we'd be swamped and she'd have to work late, and some days would be slow and she could leave early. But lately she'd been taking advantage. I appreciated the Saturday offer.

Saturday came and went and Annette never showed up. I fumed.

"We'll have another meeting," I told Terry. "I'm going to have to talk to her."

"Talk is cheap," she said. "You sure must like meetings. You have one every other day."

"Get off my case! You're always nagging me."

"Seems to me that you're upset with Annette and you're taking it out on me," she quipped.

"Don't use pop psychology on me," I snapped back.

"I'd always been taught to believe that good employees would take some of the work off of you and make your business run more smoothly and your life easier," Terry continued, undaunted. "Annette lays more work on you, screws up your business and makes your life hell. I know it's hard to let her go because you view it as a personal failure, but you are not responsible for her actions and she's got to act like an adult. She is responsible for her own actions. Make her accountable. You're taking the flack for her behavior. That dentist is right—it does reflect poorly on your clinic."

"I'll think about it," I said. Why did I keep backing off? Terry was right—I was taking this personally. I felt like I'd been a lousy manager and I was the failure, not Annette. Getting rid of her would admit my defeat. My stomach hurt. I hadn't had anything to eat all day. But I wasn't hungry.

On Monday, Annette was late, as usual. Promises, promises. Catherine was in the business office, working on the computer. She was a very good worker. I was pleased. She never missed a trick.

Annette finally showed up, fifteen minutes late. I smiled to myself when I saw Catherine glance at her watch, then toss Annette a dirty look. She was working out well. Very conscientious.

A few minutes later, I heard voices raised. It sounded like Catherine and Annette. Should I intervene? Were their voices loud enough to carry to treatment rooms? A phone call interrupted my worries. As I put down the receiver, Catherine was standing in the doorway.

"Dr. Joseph, may I have a word with you?" My watch read 12:20.

"Certainly."

We sat down in my office and Catherine sat up straight as a ramrod. She stared me in the eye.

"I know that I'm new here, but I'd like you to know that it's very distracting trying to get any work done sitting next to Annette. She likes to talk and I have a hard time concentrating. It's not the background conversations with patients; it's the conversations that she tries to draw me into. I can't talk and work at the same time. I also don't think that it's appropriate for her to be saying things about you behind your back. If she doesn't like it here, she should just leave. I've had lots of bosses I didn't like, but I always waited until I'd left the building before I said anything."

She paused. "Dr. Joseph, Annette takes Rolodex cards home. I'm not sure what she does with them, but why is she calling your patients from home after work? Do you have her working on a special project?"

I felt my eyes widen. I shook my head. "Thank you, Catherine. I'll take care of it. Why don't you take off for lunch?"

I was getting pretty hungry myself. I checked the cash box for spare change because I wanted to treat myself to a bagel. What was that white thing sticking out from underneath the cash box? I lifted it up and saw a couple checks. What were those doing there?

I pulled out the entire drawer, and checks began to cascade to the floor. Pink checks with Holly Hobby dolls. Green checks with mallards. Rainbow checks. Waterfall checks. Corporate checks. Some of the dates on them were old—months old. What was going on here? Was it true, that Annette really did think that chiropractic was a bunch of hocus pocus, that my patients would get better on their own and that there was no need for them to pay?

I called up the patient with the Holly Hobby checks. "Tina, this is Dr. Joseph. Sorry to bother you, but I have a bookkeeping question. I have a check of yours dated from two months ago that you wrote to us and it hasn't been cashed. Do you know anything about it?"

"Annette told me that I could have as many free treatments as I wanted," she replied. "But I didn't think that was right. After all, I only had small co-payments on my insurance, so it didn't hurt me financially. I always pay for any service I receive. I wouldn't dream of accepting free health care from you. I was wondering," she added, "why that check had never been cashed. You will cash it, won't you?"

"Yes, I'll cash it today, Tina. I just wanted to touch base with you. Have a nice day."

My ears were ringing. My left eye began to twitch. I'd forgotten all about running out for a bagel and grabbed the whole handful of checks, heading for my office. I heard the reception door open behind me. It was Annette. I turned on my heel and faced her. She stared, incredulous, at the pile of checks clenched in my fist.

"In my office," I growled.

"I was too busy," she blurted, as she sat across from me.

"There's no excuse for this," I countered. "You just told me the other day that you weren't too busy. Why did you tell me that? You are supposed to make deposits every day. If you can't, then find someone who will. But you don't just stick the checks in a drawer and let them rot. It screws up my bookkeeping, my patients' personal accounts, and the insurance filings. I am so disappointed in you. Between this, all your time on the phone on personal calls, phoning patients at home because you think I've billed them for services they haven't received, all the days you've come in late, and then you promised me you'd make up your time on Saturday morning and you never showed up. . .I am so disappointed. And I'm furious."

Suddenly, her eyes flashed. "So what are you going to do," she said, fluttering her heavily made-up lids. "Fire me?"

"Yes."

She blanched.

I scribbled some figures on a piece of scratch paper, then pulled out the checkbook. I made out the last check I would ever give to Annette. It totalled $35.

She frowned. "I wrote a check for severance pay for the next two weeks," I explained. "Then, I subtracted all the time you missed in the past two weeks. That's the grand total."

Her cheeks burned. Despite it all, she made a graceful exit.

CHAPTER 37

"I'm so miserable without you, it's almost like having you here."

Stephen Bishop, Song Title

It had been two weeks since Annette's departure. Despite every-thing, I missed her. It wasn't anything I could explain to my wife or, certainly, my associates. They were happy to see her go. They said that my attitude had changed and I was much less stressed out. Which was true. But it was like having my little sister move out of the house. After all we'd been through, I couldn't hate her. I felt like a mentor. I felt somehow responsible for this lost soul who would probably wander through life never really grasp what it was all about.

I missed her. Others began to miss her, as well. But for other reasons.

"Is Annette still with your office?" asked Mike, the automotive specialist.

"No," I replied. "She's no longer with us."

"I didn't think so. That's why I came back. Boy, am I glad you got rid of her."

I was in the middle of a re-exam and was trying to concentrate on a couple of orthopedic tests. Mike put a lot of pressure on his lower back by bending under the hoods of cars, twisting in all sorts of odd positions. "I noticed that you hadn't been in for a while. I thought you'd gotten busy and just couldn't fit us into your schedule," I said.

"It was more like she couldn't fit me into her schedule," said Mike, stiffening in pain as I stretched out his left leg. "She's a nice looking lady, and I was seeing her a lot at the front desk, so I asked her out. She said yes. We had dinner, saw a movie. Then she asked me back to her place. I spent the night. It was great."

He winked at me and sighed, shaking his head. Despite himself, he was grinning.

"When I left that morning, I told her I'd call her and we'd go out to eat that night. So I called her but she said she was busy. What about the next night? She said sure. I called her at the end of the day to verify the time, and she said she was busy. She asked me out to lunch for the next day. When I stopped by to pick her up, she was gone. Later, she'd said something had come up. That went on for a couple of weeks, and I finally got the hint. It was just a one-night stand and I was expecting more. She seemed like such a nice lady. So I quit calling your office. Period. I didn't care if I was in pain. And then this week, the pain got so bad, I just had to call. And I noticed that someone else answered the phone. I'm really relieved. It made me nervous to come in for my appointments and have to look at her and know that she'd used me like that."

I didn't say anything. There wasn't anything I could say.

Later that afternoon, Roger came by for his appointment. Roger was the maintenance supervisor for a local apartment complex. Tall and wiry, he had a great sense of humor and was a lot of fun to be with.

"I noticed that Annette doesn't work here any more," he said. "Things didn't work out?"

"Right."

"Yeah, they didn't work out with me, either."

Uh, oh. I could hear it coming.

"I got a phone call at about one in the morning from Annette. She sounded upset. She said that she'd broken a pipe or something and needed her plumbing fixed. I told her to call her own maintenance man in the morning. She said it couldn't wait. I told her to call her own maintenance man immediately. She lived in an entirely different apartment complex and I couldn't figure out why she needed me. I also wondered where she'd gotten my phone number, and then remembered that she worked at the front desk sometimes.

"Well, to make a long story short, I drove over there with my tool box and she greeted me at the door in her bathrobe. Her bathrobe wasn't tied or buttoned—it just hung open—and she didn't have anything on underneath it! I went in, and what can I say? I worked on her plumbing!"

I couldn't help but burst out laughing. Unbelievable. It was the only time I ever really lost it in front of a patient. But his *entendré* was so perfect, and so totally unexpected, I felt like I'd been thrown a one-liner by Yakov Smirnoff or Joan Rivers. If Mike hadn't told me his story, I might not have believed Roger, but this was definitely one for the record. I had to get up and walk across the room to compose myself.

"She has great plumbing, by the way," Roger added.

"So did you see each other after that?" I asked, mindful of Mike's story.

"No, except when I showed up for my appointments. I asked her out to lunch once, but she said she was busy. I thought that was a little strange. Actually, I think the whole thing is pretty strange, but I have to say that I had a lot of fun!"

When Joanne, my disc patient, came by that afternoon, I was surprised to hear her bring up Annette's name, as well.

"Annette was very concerned about my impending surgery," said Joanne. "I didn't want to have disc surgery and Annette said that I'd heal on my own. I told her that I wanted you to help me; after all, you're the expert, as well as the surgeons. I had no idea she knew that much about my case. She also told me that I didn't have to pay the bill. She called me twice, both times around 8 o'clock at night. I thought that it was awfully nice, but frankly, I was worried about her attitude. I think that receiving calls at home from a doctor's office is a great way to reassure patients, but Annette did everything but tell me to cancel. I just don't get it." She frowned.

"I don't know what to think. I didn't need the surgery, after all. Maybe she was right—I did heal on my own. But there was something about it that kind of bothered me. You know?"

"Do you mean you felt like your privacy had been invaded?" I asked.

"Yes! That's it! She was a very sweet lady, Dr. Joseph, but I'm still glad that she's not working here any more."

"Why didn't you tell me this earlier?"

"I didn't want to interfere. I thought it was some kind of a program set up by your office. I don't know."

"Joanne, next time, interfere. Please. You are the reason our clinic exists. We didn't set up practice to provide a playground for employees."

Annette's presence was like a ghost, coming back to take care of unfinished business. I couldn't shake her.

A couple of months later, I was working out at the gym and ran into Fred, Annette's red hot lover—the one Terry has said was a scum ball. "I thought you moved out of state," I said.

"I did, but things didn't work out. I decided to move back here and go back to my old job. Need a spotter?"

"Sure," I said.

Fred was a great-looking guy. No matter how sweaty he got, his hair was always perfect. The cuts in his muscles looked like they'd been sculpted from marble. Too bad he had treated Annette so badly.

"Does Annette still work for you?" he asked, lifting the barbell over my head and setting it down. He unscrewed the collars and began exchanging the weights.

"No. She's no longer with us."

"Oh. I wondered about that. I didn't think she was there any more." He paused.

"She was really a strange bird," he said, finishing up with the weights and tightening the collars again. He leaned up against the weight rack.

Uh-oh, I could hear it coming.

"She used to call me up in the middle of the night and beg me to come over and screw her. I was so tired I could hardly see straight! Then, after awhile, she just began to ignore me. I never could figure out what the problem was."

I could feel the goose bumps crawling up my arms. Was that "Twilight Zone" music that was buzzing in my ears? That was just the opposite story that Annette had passed through the office! It was Fred who had been waking up Annette for so long! We were all convinced that Fred was the lowest life form on the planet. Now, reality had once more been turned on its ear. Good thing I was lying down.

My friend the Christian counselor invited me to lunch not long after that. Before long, the subject of Annette came up.

"I'm glad that she's not working for you anymore, Vincent," he said. "She was a very mixed-up lady."

"That's putting it mildly. Do you know how many people have come up and said something to me? How come nobody told me this before?"

"It's not easy," he said. "You have your reasons for hiring and keeping people. Maybe she was really good with insurance billing or something."

I choked on a piece of lettuce. "I can sympathize with you, though, Vincent," he continued. "It's not very nice when your employees sabotage you, regardless of their motivations."

I nodded.

"You know, she had quite a reputation around town," he continued. "My wife warned me to stay away from her. She thought that people would start to talk."

"Uh, well, I was sort of wondering."

"Who, me?" He rolled his eyes and sighed. He pushed away his lunch as though it had suddenly been poisoned. "I should have known better. That's what I get for trying to be a nice guy. She just wanted to talk. She wanted guidance for her children. You know me, I'm a counselor. I tried to help her."

"That's okay," I said. "I believe you." A surprised look flashed across his face, as though I would be the last person in the world to even think for a moment that he might have succumbed to temptation. "I almost called you about that, you know. People were talking. I wanted to warn you. But then, I figured, you're an adult. You can handle your own life without my interference."

"I wish you would have called, Vincent. I had no idea that her reputation was so outrageous." Worry lines creased his forehead. He looked absolutely sick.

"You and I are about the only two people in the world she hasn't slept with," I said, trying to inject some humor into the situation. "What do you suppose she doesn't like about us?"

He roared with laughter. He even perked up enough to order dessert.

About a week later, I ran into Nancy in the supermarket. She was happy with her new job and seemed happy to see me. This time, it was I who decided to bring up the subject of Annette.

"I owe you an apology," I said. "I was told that it was Annette who was helping you with the computer, not the other way around."

Her eyes widened.

"When Annette met with you to discuss your work, did she tell you that I was upset with you?" I asked.

"Yes. I couldn't figure out why, when I was not only doing my work, but hers, as well."

"I see." Nancy looked concerned. She was beginning to catch on.

"I liked your work very much, Nancy. I didn't manage the computer system, so I had to take Annette's word for it when she said you were slow and that you didn't know the system. That's why I watched you so much. Annette is no longer with us," I continued. "I let her go. Things just got out of hand."

"Oh." Nancy's face was unreadable. At first she looked pleased. Then a look of sadness veiled her face.

"I'm sorry," I said. "I thought you two were friends."

The look of sadness deepened and I noted a little flash of anger in her eyes. "I thought so, too," she said, and wheeled her cart in the other direction.

When the report came back from the agency that brought my collections up to date, it wasn't a pretty sight. That year, we watched thousands of dollars go down the drain. It was certainly an expensive lesson to learn. It would have paid the rent for an entire year.

Now I know a smoke screen when I see one. Annette's technique was so smooth, it could have fooled Sigmund Freud himself. She had us tripping over one another, accusing each other, blaming each other, suspicious of everyone except her. I was the main scapegoat, of course. The big bad boss man always is.

I don't think anyone was as relieved to see Annette go as Terry was. Anyone who could drive a wedge of suspicion into our relationship was definitely not what we needed. And Terry knew that Annette's antics were sapping my energies and blurring my focus, which needed to be directed toward helping patients. Last but not least, Terry was furious and nearly despondent over the money that had been lost. Anyone who has ever been in business for himself knows how hard it is to stay afloat. Imagine what it would be like to discover the repercussions from an employee like Annette.

Annette hadn't actually taken any of the money. She'd just re-routed it. And never collected it to begin with. Because it took so many months to straighten out our files, we zeroed out the balances of those dozens of patients who were never billed by Annette. We had to. We couldn't blindside patients over a year later with bills for hundreds of dollars, months after they'd assumed everything had been paid by insurance.

I didn't press charges. How do you press charges for incompetence? For lunacy? Although I considered suing for slander because of the insurance rumors, my attorney advised me to leave bad enough alone and write the whole thing off at the end of the year. He said it just wasn't worth it. I cracked down on late insurance billings and kept a close watch on companies that didn't pay when they were supposed to. I still treated some people for free—a generosity my wife bemusedly calls a character flaw. Sometimes my patients with a cash flow problem repaid me with food or handmade items or a book or auto repair work.

Helping out in the community, giving to charities, treating indigent patients who respond well to my care—that's the nice part of being a doctor. It's a lot more fulfilling than pulling open a desk drawer and finding a pile of very old, uncashed checks, and dealing with an out-of-control employee hell-bent on sabotage.

CHAPTER 38

"Any fool can make a rule."

Henry David Thoreau

Months before the baby was due, Terry and I had discussed dos and don'ts regarding childbirth and baby care in the hospital. Vitamin K shots were fine. But no erythromycin in the eyes. (The antibiotic now commonly replaces the more caustic silver nitrate.)

Terry was allergic to nearly every antibiotic in existence—and she didn't want the baby exposed needlessly. Certainly there was no need for the drops, considering they were given in order to protect the infant from blindness due to venereal disease during the child's journey through the birth canal.

The obstetrician said fine. Terry asked that it be put in writing. He suggested she talk to the head nurse in the nursery. The head nurse at the nursery said that it was all right with her as long as Terry talked with the obstetrician.

After fourteen hours of labor and somewhere around thirty-four stitches, Terry was ready for bed, I was cuddling the baby, and the obstetrician was ready to call it a day. All the baby needed was to be weighed and given the vitamin K shot.

Not so fast. The pediatrician on call was refusing to treat the newborn. Eh? It's against the law to refuse E-mycin. He didn't want to get tangled up in any legal mess.

What about the hospital patient's bill of rights? What about informed consent? What about all the discussions before the baby was born?

No go. It was 10 P.M. and no one would touch the baby. Word was sent out for a pediatrician who would take care of the situation.

After many phone calls, a pediatrician was located. But before he would agree to forgo the eye drops, Terry had to be tested for gonorrhea—because the doctor didn't want any problems should the baby turn out blind. Sort of an "I told you so" precautionary measure.

We were mighty upset. The obstetrician wasn't too thrilled, either. He wanted to go home. We were so thrilled with the whole experience, with all its wonder, pain, fascination and hard work, that a gonorrhea test really marred the euphoria. We didn't need this. We were young and elated and our baby was perfect. Couldn't we just relax and enjoy this special time? The baby was weighed, placed under lights for a bit of jaundice, and given a vitamin K shot. Then a nurse cornered me.

"Why don't you want E-mycin drops?" she asked.

"Because it's treatment without a diagnosis," I said. "My wife doesn't have a venereal disease. Neither do I. We don't sleep around. Never have. So why give a drug for no reason?"

"But what if something happens?"

"Like what? Nothing will happen. Unless the baby contracts something from the hospital." The nurse raised an eyebrow and frowned. "Somebody came up with this law because he saw a lot of babies going blind because the mothers were transmitting infections during delivery. Therefore, every mother giving birth is guilty until proven innocent. What kind of logic is that? It makes me mad. The government has no right to tell me what kind of health care I should have. I have the right to say no to any type of drug or surgery. The government thinks it can take that away."

"No one else has ever questioned it. Why should you? The people who make those laws know what they're doing."

"No, they don't. That's why I get involved in politics. You should too. This is one state law that I am going to work to unmake." This woman had absolutely no interest in what was best for our baby and absolutely every intention of keeping her job and maintaining the status quo. She made me sick.

Having run out of arguments, the nurse proceeded to the nursery, where I stood over her and the other nurses for well over an hour. They tried their best to get rid of me.

"Aren't you getting tired? You should be with your wife."

"No, I shouldn't. I should be with the baby. The obstetrician is with my wife."

"Don't you want to go home and get some sleep?"

"No."

"Aren't you hungry?"

"No."

"You don't have to stay here the whole time."

"Yes, I do."

"You don't trust us."

"You got that right."

"How can you say that?"

"Because you argued with me in the hallway and made faces in the delivery room. And I overheard you talking together."

"We're not going to do anything."

"I'm not leaving."

"You're not really supposed to be here. It's only for doctors and nurses."

"I'm a doctor."

They rolled their eyes.

A month later, when nearly a hundred dollars in extra charges for unnecessary gonorrhea blood tests showed up on the hospital bill, we vowed to change the law that assumed everyone in the state had an untreated, undiagnosed venereal disease.

We're still working on it.

CHAPTER 39

"When they first brought the baby in to her. . .she stared, inert, and thought, This is the author of my pain."

Bessie Brueur, The Actress

She lumbered down the hallway, her feet rustling softly on the carpeting, her shoulders occasionally grazing the walls. Her cheeks glowed, her eyes sparkled, her hair shone. But her lips were taut, her expression grim. She settled down on the treatment table with a great sigh.

"I can't wait until this is over with. I've got a whole month to go."

"You'll be surprised at how fast the time goes," I said. "Before you know it, you'll be surrounded by cards and flowers and nursing your first baby."

"None of my friends ever complained about their backs like this," she said.

"Not everyone is the same," I replied. "You're going to work every day and you're sitting long hours. You need to get up and stretch every half hour. The baby is putting a lot of pressure on your spine. A professor of mine once said that in the evolution of the human body, the lower spine hasn't quite made it yet. When you prick your finger, you can locate the source of pain immediately. But when you've got pain in your lower back, it just feels like the whole area is on fire."

"That's for sure."

"Let's put you face down on the table." I had a drop piece for pregnant women. It eased open to allow room for Georgi's ample belly. I gave her a good stretch by placing one hand on her pelvic area and one hand on her mid back. She was tense and her muscles were tight. Her skin felt warm to the touch—much warmer than my other patients, but that was to be expected.

Since she'd gotten so big, I couldn't adjust her in side posture any more, so I adjusted her from the back. She experienced a great deal of relief, but she had a couple of nasty trigger points in her lumbar region.

"I have a little something you can take home." I handed her a brand new TENS unit. "This is a transdermal electrical neurostimulator. You apply this gel to the little pads, then place them on the areas that need it the most. You can control the intensity with this dial. It blocks the nerves to the area and gives you pain relief."

"Won't this hurt the baby?"

"You're not going to put it on the baby, you're going to put it on your back."

"Can I use it on other parts of my body, like my calves?"

"Sure, but most people use it on their lower backs because they can tuck the unit in the back of their pants or carry it in a pocket. If you use it anywhere else, you've got to sit or lie down. It's very safe. And the best part is that you won't be tempted to take aspirin for pain while you're using it, and you know that you're not supposed to take aspirin, especially the closer you get to delivery."

She nodded. So far, she didn't have any permanent damage to her lower back from the pregnancy. If she continued to stretch, and put up her feet as often as possible, she'd be fine.

Diane, a sales rep who spent the entire nine months of her pregnancy running from client to client and hopping on jets up and down the East Coast, ended up with arthritis in her ankles. She also had a compressed disc in her lower spine, which I could help but not totally reverse. She saw me only for crisis care and ignored every last bit of my advice. It took her two years to recover from her experience, and she decided not to have any more children. I felt bad, because I felt certain that if she'd taken more time to put up her feet and visit the clinic for adjustments, she could have had a couple more kids without too much trouble.

But Georgi was playing it smart, and I knew she'd be fine. She'd been referred by her OB/GYN and I knew that in all other respects she was doing well and the baby was progressing perfectly.

"I'm going to refer you to a massage therapist every ten days," I said. "It will make you feel a lot better. Not only will it help your back, but it will help the circulation in your legs, too. It's not uncommon for women to have swelling and end up with spider veins or even varicose veins because of pregnancy."

I brought her husband into the treatment room and showed him where to apply pressure on the cushiony part of Georgi's lower back next to the spine if she had back labor. He practiced it a few times, but I had to tell him to push harder. "I don't want to hurt her," he said.

"Don't worry about that," I laughed, remembering my own experience in the delivery room. "Just trust your instincts. And your thumb is going to get tired, so curl your fingers and use your knuckles."

The older woman I treated immediately after Georgi scowled and wagged a knobby finger at me. "Shame on you for treating a pregnant woman," she said. "I saw you go in that room. That's not safe."

"What?" I said. "Who told you that?"

"My doctor told me that when I was pregnant—and I have five healthy children."

That was 150 years ago, I thought, but I held my tongue.

"I get lots of referrals from obstetricians for low back pain," I said. The old woman gasped and threw her hand to her chest. "What are things coming to?"

"It makes sense," I said. "I'm sure you suffered from back pain when you were pregnant. Now look at you—arthritis, no mobility in your joints at all, and you've got hypoplasia, where your spine didn't develop correctly and the change in your posture during pregnancy made it worse. Chiropractic adjustments would have helped you immensely during your pregnancies. The fact that you come in to my office for treatments now indicates that you think they're safe."

"Yes, but I'm not pregnant, my dear!"

In a last-ditch effort, I gave her a brochure explaining chiropractic adjustments during pregnancy. Sometimes another source, particularly a written source, held more credibility than a friend or relative, or even a doctor.

"Well, look at this!" she exclaimed, pointing to a photo of a pregnant woman lying face down on a table with a drop piece. "You never told me you had these gadgets! I thought you just put those poor ladies flat on their bellies!"

I broke out laughing. Lucky for me, she laughed, too.

Georgi delivered an eight-pound boy three weeks later. He had a head full of hair and a yell that could shatter your eardrums. She was the happiest mother I'd ever seen. Much of it, I suspect, was relief; she really did want to get the whole thing over with. She stopped by for a treatment a week after the delivery. "That TENS unit saved my life," she commented, returning it to me. "It was my best friend the whole week before the baby came. You should tell all your patients to use this thing."

I put her on the treatment table and ignored the drop piece. "My stomach!" she cried. "I'm flat on my stomach! It feels so good!"

Even though her face was buried in the headrest, I knew that she was smiling all the way through the treatment.

CHAPTER 40

"The only normal people are the ones you don't know very well."

Joe Ancis

Laurie came to see me after she'd been rear-ended in her '89 Supra. She had a wicked case of whiplash. She'd been the usual route—emergency room, half a dozen M.D.s, pain killers. She'd heard that chiropractic could solve all her problems. Friends had said that people could be healed in just one day.

That's the kind of patient who gives chiropractors the creeps. Wave that wand, shake those rattles and voilà! A magical cure. Made me suspicious, too. Sure, it was an ego trip, but she was really messed up from the accident, so saying that she had unrealistic expectations was an understatement. This therapy was going to take a long, long time.

Nevertheless, she passed all the malingerer tests. I never stooped so low as to throw a dollar bill on the floor to observe the suddenly limber patient enthusiastically pick it up and then say, "Oops—guess I'm not as sore as I thought!" but there are subtle things that doctors do.

Laurie was barely eighteen years old. She was accompanied by her mother during her first chiropractic visit. Turned out that Laurie's dad had run off with some young thing and left his family in the lurch while he caroused in California.

Laurie chased after him and thrived on the surfing and partying she indulged herself in while in Newport Beach. But, soon enough, the unwanted daughter was sent home. Her dad had a new life and didn't need remnants of the past asking him for drinking money and car keys. It was his turn to do all that, now that he'd hit mid-life crisis.

Dejected, betrayed, lonely and scared, she resented having to live in the blue-collar military and shipbuilding city of Newport News, Virginia. She was bored. And, most of all, she repeatedly made mention of the fact that she hated living in the Bible Belt.

I wasn't Laurie's first chiropractor. She had made an appointment with the chiropractor down the street. But she said that it scared her to have her neck cracked. And besides, she said that the doctor had stared at her breasts just like all the other doctors did. They were all male chauvinist pigs.

Although she had a gorgeous, full head of hair, its color changed monthly. Once it was jet black. The next time it was orange—a nasty case of chronic hair syndrome. She wore enough makeup to keep the cosmetics industry indefinitely holding its own on the Dow Jones Industrial Average.

Her eyes were out of this world. Literally. She had somehow managed to find a pair of eerie blue contact lenses with colored lines that radiated from her pupils like the spokes in a wheel. Her fingernails were day-glow orange talons one day, black the next.

And she was dressed to kill. Nighttime attire was her favorite. And the cleavage, well, that was another story altogether.

So I stared straight into her otherworldly eyes and talked about my wife. A lot.

So far, so good. Laurie continued her care, even allowing me to adjust her neck. Which was great, because her neck was in rough shape. As was her ego. Every adjustment was an emotional experience. Tears and tales of woe. On and on.

Since I seemed oblivious to Laurie's cleavage, her personality seemed to take a turn for the worse. Or better. Depending.

She said she had dropped out of high school and was going straight to college to major in accounting. Said she had a lot of smarts. But the next week, she said she'd been accepted to medical school. No telling where her talents would take her.

I didn't bat an eyelash. Just kept going on with those adjustments. Frankly, I was pretty pleased that I'd gotten the swelling down. She had good rotation in her joints now. Lots of good movement. No more stiffness. The pain was much better.

But Laurie had headaches, which meant that I had to take a detailed history to get at their etiology. "Is there anything you can think of that triggers your headaches?" I asked.

"Yes," she replied. "Sometimes they happen when I have sex. My boyfriend likes rough sex. That's okay with me. I like the idea." But when push came to shove, literally, she was out of her league. She broke a fingernail. Tsk, tsk.

But wait—there was more. More sex. And more details. Oral sex hurt her neck. Laurie rubbed her neck, arched her back, and ran her tongue around her lips to illustrate precisely how this all worked. She explained how she tried the traditional missionary style, but that hurt her lower back. "You understand, don't you, Dr. Joseph?"

I was getting pretty good at tuning out her chatter and concentrating on her adjustments. I knew that she was trying to impress me. She was arching her back and waiting for my reaction. "Hmmm, that doesn't surprise me one bit," I said.

As far as her adjustments were concerned, I was pretty pleased. Her neck had now achieved its full range of motion. Not a single kink. I just wished I could say that for her mind. I still believed that she wasn't a malingerer. She wasn't making up her symptoms. But she was hysterical—the symptoms she had were overblown.

At that point, her attorney was getting antsy to settle the case and collect as much money as possible from her car accident. He wanted her referred to a surgeon. He didn't like chiropractors. But Laurie wasn't really interested in talking about it. She wanted to tell me that she had a part time job as a bookkeeper. And she really wanted to get married and have babies. If her boyfriend wouldn't marry her, then she'd just have his baby anyway. If she could only get pregnant.

I'd had just about enough. I decided she needed counseling. My working diagnosis and treatment was hampered by the fact that every time she opened her mouth, I presumed it would be another goofy story, and I had no way of telling which of her symptoms were real and which were fabricated for my benefit.

A few weeks back, I'd dealt with a case of child abuse that I'd referred to the family minister and was pleased that it had been handled so well. Since a lot of people are afraid of psychiatrists and counselors, ministers are usually a safe bet. If it worked once, it would work again, right?

That was the critical mistake that every young doctor makes.

"Do you go to church?" I asked.

"Sort of," she replied. She started to look uncomfortable.

"Do you know a minister?" I prodded.

"Yes." She refused to meet my eyes. Her breath was becoming shallow.

"I think, in light of your problems, it would help to see a minister. Just to talk about things. Chiropractic philosophy dictates that your body should not be broken up into separate units," I said. "There's the physical aspect, the emotional and spiritual aspect and the nutritional aspect. If you don't address all of those, you aren't being treated properly. We've already addressed nutrition and the physical end of things. Let's try the emotional and spiritual approach."

Laurie seemed a little surprised by this. Apparently her minister didn't do counseling in the same manner in which the good doctor was accustomed. She would enlighten me.

With a deep breath and a rather condescending air, made somewhat more irritating by the drumming of her exceptionally long, painted, black fingernails, she began to explain her lifestyle and philosophy. First of all, she said, her minister wasn't a graduate of any divinity school that anyone had ever heard of. Because he was a satanic warlock. And she was a witch. And she told me that she had killed people. And the reason she really wanted to get married and have kids was so she could sacrifice her baby.

She talked up a storm for a good half hour. I knew I had other patients waiting, and twice I was buzzed on the intercom, but, mesmerized, I listened closely to tales that would make many folks turn tail and run for the nearest church. A couple of times, I found myself mentally repeating, "It's only a movie; it's only a movie," but after a while it lost its effect.

As a scientist at heart, I like to save judgment until all the evidence is in. But that doesn't mean I can't indulge myself by actually enjoying the data. I'd never had a patient who was so intent upon manipulating me and who came so close—I alternately felt anger, sorrow, confusion, and flat-out fascination.

Even before she'd finished, I'd already begun to form my theory. Although I had made the mistake of assuming that since counseling from a minister worked in one case, it would work again, I was not so impressionable to make the mistake of becoming emotionally shell-shocked. I decided to trust my gut response.

What I heard was not the sordid, grisly tale of a seasoned murderer. What I heard was a rejected little girl crying out for attention, spinning any yarn that would cause me to gasp.

Laurie came pretty close to hitting the nail on the head. I recalled that her first attempt at attention-getting was to give me the poor-poor-pitiful-me story. When that didn't work, she poured on the sex appeal. I countered that by telling her I was a family man. Big into education. Down on drugs. She countered that with talk about getting into medical school. Or was it accounting school? Or engineering?

None of that worked, either. So she tried a last-ditch effort, one that was guaranteed to shock the most hardened Bible-Belt Christian from complacency.

Except that I wasn't a Bible-Belt devotee. I was a Yankee. Not totally corrupt—just worldly enough. Jesus said to be as wise as serpents and as innocent as doves. I'd seen the strip joints in St. Paul that were closed down by a shrewd City Council member who used to ply her trade as a prostitute. I'd passed by the gay bars on Minneapolis' Hennepin Avenue. Uptown Minneapolis was littered with little shops with purple and silver curtains where women with obscenely long fingernails read tea leaves and sold crystals for astronomical amounts of money. The best of Minnesota is its shimmering lakes, miles of pine trees, rolling landscapes dotted with peacefully grazing cows. The Twin Cities boast opera, fine arts, booming business and architecture to die for. But that's only part of the picture.

I'll admit I'm pretty naive. And I look young. I was pegged as an easy target. Sacrificing babies would surely do it. I spent so much time talking about my wife, after all. During Laurie's treatment, in her mind I'd alternately played father, brother, lover, doctor, and finally, adversary.

Now all the pieces came together: The Twilight Zone eyes, freeze-dried hair, aversion to the Bible Belt. Laurie probably did believe in witchcraft. But a murderer? No chance.

One day soon after, I was having lunch with a medical doctor on the other side of town, a guy I palled around with from time to time. I mentioned Laurie's story to the doctor and was totally unprepared for the response. "Stay away from her! You don't know what you're getting yourself into! She's dangerous!" The guy went berserk—really thought we were all in danger.

I was pretty surprised. And disgusted. This was a side of my buddy that I'd never seen before. I could just picture him sitting in the front row of a movie theater watching *The Exorcist* like a little boy with wide eyes, taking it all in, believing every last bit of it. I clamped my mouth shut and never brought up the subject again. It wasn't just that my colleague was so superstitious; it was that he was so lacking in compassion. All I could do was shake my head. I knew that I was going to eventually lose Laurie as a patient, and I worried about her future. But I felt a sadness somewhere inside, too, for the friendship that I'd just seen disappear before my eyes with a colleague that I really didn't know at all.

Laurie's boyfriend had talked to me about how he wanted to be hypnotized to be a better bodybuilder. And he wanted more discipline on his diet. Since Laurie seemed to lean in the direction of the mystical anyway, I thought that hypnotism might just be the way to go. And I knew just the right person. Not only was she a hypnotist, but she was a Christian psychologist. But Laurie didn't know that. She took me up on my offer.

Laurie visited the psychologist twice before she gave up on that, too.

Then Laurie's attorney got back into the act. He made her drive all the way to Richmond to get a second opinion from an orthopedic surgeon. The surgeon wanted to operate on the occipital muscles.

I suggested yet another opinion. I knew she wasn't a surgery candidate. But the lawyer was getting hot. And he was running Laurie's life.

During all this, Laurie's neck was suddenly getting worse. She had called her dad several times and he refused to return her phone calls. She was getting more and more depressed.

In disgust and desperation, I played my last card. I told the attorney all about Laurie's tales of witches and warlocks and baby killing. "If you put her on the stand," I said, "she'll be an incredibly unreliable witness. One minute she's telling people she's going to medical school, the next, she's a bookkeeper. And if she doesn't ruin her own case, I'll do it for her. I'll blow the case wide open. It doesn't matter whether or not anyone believes her fabricated tales about devil worship. The point is, with her history of tall tales, no jury will ever get the facts straight about the car accident. Period."

The lawyer suddenly saw my point. He told her to see a psychiatrist. And she went. The doctor put her on medication. And then Laurie broke up with her boyfriend—decided she didn't want kids, anyway.

I cut Laurie's visits down as her neck improved. And one day, it suddenly occurred to me that I'd lost track of her. I tried calling her at home, but her phone was disconnected. I couldn't get hold of any of her relatives, particularly her mother.

It was a sad ending for an unusual case. I had to remind myself that there were just some people I couldn't help.

Several weeks later, I ran into Laurie at a local restaurant. Her hair was a normal shade of blonde. She wasn't wearing quite as much makeup. Her fingernails were shorter and an acceptable shade of pink. She told me that her neck felt much better. Overall, her entire attitude seemed to have improved. But I couldn't help but notice that she was really hustling—so many men, so little time.

Pleased with her progress, I ventured a little further. "What are you doing with your career?" I inquired. I held my breath.

"Oh, haven't I told you?," she said breathily, quite obviously pleased with herself. "I'm running for President."

CHAPTER 41

"A woman is always a fickle, unstable thing."

Virgil, *Aeneid*

Patricia was being seen in the clinic for neck pain and lower back pain resulting from a car accident. She'd enlisted in the Army a couple of years before and specialized in computer programming.

I don't normally pay all that much attention to my patients' looks, but Patricia was like a pink polka-dotted elephant in the middle of my otherwise conservative clinic. You couldn't help but notice her. Tall, square-shouldered, slim-hipped, she would have made a perfect swim team member. Except that she didn't like to swim. It would have ruined her makeup. She always wore makeup, accenting her almond-shaped eyes and highlighting her cheekbones. I knew that she wore waterproof mascara because, after lying face down on a treatment table for twenty minutes at a stretch, she arose as polished as she'd been the moment she walked in. She wore her hair curled to her shoulders and frizzed above her forehead. Her perfume lingered long after she'd left the room. According to all the television commercials and magazine ads, perfume that lingers is sexy and alluring. But to an asthmatic, it's hell. Especially those perfume inserts in the ladies' magazines.

As a man, I would never waste that much time on my looks, and I am always baffled by women who assign it such priority.

Patricia's choice of attire was distinctly upper-class and inappropriately sexy. I had no idea that people who enlisted in the military made so much money. I noticed Neiman Marcus labels on her sweaters. When she donned a clinic gown and stretched herself out on a treatment table, Frederick's of Hollywood labels on her brilliant pink lace underwear were prominent. One afternoon, she sauntered in wearing an eye-stopping little black dress that sported a V-neck halfway to Neptune. What she would wear to her next office visit became the topic of the day for the front desk staff on several occasions.

I'd only treated Patricia a couple of times when she ended up being seen by Dr. Dillard because I was called out of the office. She complained about him to the staff, but her complaints were vague. Since no one could pinpoint the problem, Patricia continued to see him. Then, one day, he called in sick and I ended up treating Patricia.

She didn't want to be treated by me, either. I was thoroughly confused. What had I done wrong? She fussed and sighed and then suddenly giggled while I took her blood pressure (she'd complained of dizziness and I wanted to rule out any other sources). Her blood pressure was unbelievably high, and her pulse was racing. I waited a few moments, then checked again. Her pulse had slowed down, then suddenly picked up. "Your blood pressure is high," I said, "and your pulse is erratic."

She smiled slowly and said, "it's always like that when I'm here."

Well, doctors' offices make some people nervous, I rationalized.

Then I used my ophthalmoscope to examine her eyes. Close-up eye exams are uncomfortable for a lot of patients because it's no fun having someone shine a very bright light deep into your eye when you're forced not to blink. On top of it, you have to get up very close and really invade the patient's space. Even shy people can handle having their backs worked on, because backs are so impersonal. After all, short of walking away, turning your back on someone is the most impersonal thing you can do. But faces. . .faces are personal. And this time, I was the one who was uncomfortable. Patricia had no qualms at all about being a half-inch away from my face. She seemed to be enjoying it. I could hear her breathing, and the breaths came so close together that it almost sounded like panting. I thought it was pretty strange, but I decided to focus on the eye exam. Something odd was going on deep inside her eye. And her pupils weren't contracting properly. I began to wonder if I should refer her out.

"I may have to re-examine you," I said. "You seem to be having some complications."

"Oh, please do," she smiled. The words were more a caress than a comment. The hairs on the back of my neck began to stand up, reminding me of the vampire movies that my parents used to let me stay up late to watch on weekends.

Her demeanor abruptly shifted and she sat up as though her commanding officer had just walked in the room. The change startled me. It was inappropriate. Her behavior was disjointed. Combined with erratic physical findings, I began to wonder if she was on medication but hadn't told me.

But my musings were interrupted when she slid quickly off the exam table. She pulled herself up to her impressive 5'6", 36-24-36 frame, snapped to attention and stared me square in the eye. "I want you to refer me to another chiropractor because it makes me nervous to be around you," she said. "I have a crush on you. You make me hot."

She breathed through her nose and I could see her nostrils flare.

"I'd be happy to refer you out," I told her, in my most businesslike tone, "but you've only got four more treatments left. Is it really worth it?"

She tilted her chin and continued to stare at me, this time at an angle. "Fine. I'll do my best to deal with it," she said.

I credit myself for being an intelligent man. I've spotted all sorts of bizarre illnesses that would make great entries in any juried medical or chiropractic journal. But could I spot someone on the make if she were right under my nose? Someone who deliberately dressed up to catch my attention and chose her underwear with the same amount of care I would allow when analyzing an x-ray?

As fate would have it, I lifted weights three times a week with her husband. Soon to be ex-husband, I might add. He was employed by the gym and basically lived at the place. Patricia had told me on more than one occasion that her husband had had numerous affairs. Looking back on it, I should have picked up on the innuendo: "He's having affairs, ergo, I have permission, as well."

But that wasn't the story I was getting from Charles. "I met a really nice lady here last week, Vincent," he told me. "I'm wondering if I should ask her out. Do you think that would be something I should do if my divorce isn't finalized yet?"

Patricia was constantly complaining about her husband's spending habits. She told me that he bought clothes hand-over-fist, drove an expensive sports car, and ate at only the most exclusive restaurants. Now I really began to wonder if she wasn't on drugs. Charles drove a battered 1985 Mustang. He wore only old, sweaty, torn T-shirts and running shorts to the gym. And he toted his lunch in a brown paper bag. One day after he'd messed up on nearly every set he tried at the gym, he sat on a bench and hung his head in his hands. He ran his fingers through his short, sweaty hair with brisk, irritated gestures. He was in great shape, so I knew that his problems at the gym had nothing to do with strength.

"There's a lot of spending going on," he said, "but it's not me. She's always out shopping. She suffers from depression and I guess it makes her feel better. But then when the bills come, it makes her even more depressed because we have no way to pay them. She's on drugs, Vince. She's dealing and using on base."

Ah, so that's where the money came from, I thought. I knew that enlisted military folks weren't loaded. That explained her physical findings, too. I shook my head. Charles seemed like such a nice guy.

And naive, too. How did he saddle himself with this woman? I wondered how he'd feel if he knew she'd been coming on to me. I was certainly in no hurry to find out.

The next time Patricia came to the clinic for a treatment, she told me that her divorce papers had all been signed. Clara fiddled with the electrical stim equipment over in the corner while I deflected comments from Patricia.

"That's it," she said. "The divorce is final. We met at 4:00." She smiled up at me, inviting a comment. I made none.

That night, I ran into Charles at the gym. "I heard your divorce was finalized today. That must have been really rough."

"Huh? You kidding? I've been working here all day. Don't I *wish* it were final! Where did you get that idea?"

"Uh, never mind." But he knew.

"The best thing that could happen to me would be to sign those papers," said Charles. "I'm planning on moving to Nebraska but I can't go until we finish the divorce. Patricia doesn't know that," he added.

"If Patricia is so flaky and so undependable and on drugs," I asked, "surely it must show in her work. Why doesn't the Army kick her out?"

"Because she hasn't been tested for drugs, and she's the only one who knows the computer system."

An eloquent example of good luck and making oneself indispensable at work, I thought.

I certainly wasn't expecting Patricia to re-injure herself. She was out walking her very spoiled and very aggressive Akita, when he decided to walk her. He dragged her through the mud and over the curb before she decided that it would be in her best interest to let go of the leash. Patricia came in the clinic with bruises from head to toe. They were extremely evident given that she'd chosen to wear a little sleeveless, v-neck, crepe mini-skirt number.

We came up with a new treatment plan that would take about four weeks. Much of it involved ice and adjustments to just about every joint in her body. The most important part of the treatment plan involved signing up her dog for obedience school.

I told her that unless she was willing to train her dog, her office visits with me would be a waste of time, because she would be continually re-injuring herself. As I said aloud the words "waste of time," it suddenly occurred to me that she would be happy to have any excuse to see me, any time of the day or night. As if reading my mind, she stared straight into my eyes and said, "You have very kissable lips."

That was it. I thought that I'd handled it before by talking about my wife and baby, but it was evident that I'd lost control of the patient. I'd read an article recently in a malpractice insurance pamphlet about this type of thing. The consultants suggested A) Do not have any sexual relationship with an individual who is still a patient; B) Always bring a staff member into the treatment room as a witness; C) If the situation worsens, refer the patient to another doctor. I'd already implemented steps one and two; it caused me no heartburn to move on to step three and ask her to leave. It was a big relief.

Patricia was already familiar with the chiropractor down the road, so I sent her on her way, and I mailed her file and x-rays to that clinic. She was expecting it. She was almost victorious, in a smug sort of way. "See, I'm just too much for you, huh, doc?" she seemed to say as she pursed her lips and tottered away on heels that were much too high for her to handle and certainly bad for her spine. She reminded me of a little girl playing dress-up in her mother's clothes. . .except that she filled them out awfully well.

I felt sorry for her. I felt a little sorry for myself, too. Couldn't someone normal have a crush on me? Just once?

CHAPTER 42

"When I go to the beauty parlor, I always use the emergency exit.
Sometimes I just go for an estimate."

Phyllis Diller

Keeping a doctor's office clean is not difficult if you are the type who pays attention to details. Keep the wastepaper baskets emptied. Clean up kids' candy wrappers from the waiting room. Keep the magazines in order. Make sure the cold packs are cold and the hot packs are hot. Make sure the exam tables always have clean paper.

Sometimes it's easier to remember to clean up. Like when someone leaves a really big mess. Or an imprint.

Mrs. Beasley was a little on the plump side. Jolly, happy-go-lucky, and wealthy. She loved her gold jewelry and her makeup. She loved to chat about making cookies for her grandchildren and shopping at the most exclusive stores in town. But, oh, shopping was so tedious. It hurt her back. She really needed an adjustment on her upper back. She carried her suitcase-size purse on her shoulder and it strained her muscles and caused her to favor one side. So she lay on the table and put her face in the head rest—the kind of head rest that has a big space in the middle for your nose.

When she sat up, Mrs. Beasley's face was still on the headrest. At least, that's what it looked like. And since the paper was divided to leave room for her nose, the imprint was a perfect profile: lipstick, blush, eye shadow and mascara.

My mischievous streak surfaces every now and then. After Mrs. Beasley left, I carefully removed the headrest paper and placed it in a bag. I knew that my wife would be happy to help me in my effort.

"How would you like to do a little art project?" I asked Terry when I got home that night. Terry immediately assumed I was going to commission her to do a poster for the local health club or a flyer for a patient appreciation day at the clinic. Not even close.

I removed the headrest paper from the bag and held it up. "What do you think this is?" Well, she of course knew it was the imprint of a person's face.

"Boy, does she wear a lot of makeup," Terry said.

"I want to play a joke on her. How about if you connect the dots? Just draw a line for her forehead and nose and outline the eye a little?"

Terry blushed. "Won't she get mad? What if she doesn't have a sense of humor? I don't want to be responsible for a lost patient."

"Trust me—I'm a doctor."

So the dirty deed was done and it was beautiful. I laughed so hard I cried. I couldn't wait for Mrs. Beasley's next visit.

The day dawned bright and cheerful and Mrs. Beasley was her rosy-cheeked self, literally. "I have a present for you," I said. "My wife is an artist and she made you something." Mrs. Beasley glowed with anticipation.

I ceremoniously unfolded the headrest paper-cum-portrait and held it up for Mrs. Beasley. She squinted a little, trying to make out the image. She looked confused as she reached for the object. I felt deflated as her non-reaction sank in.

"I'm really sorry," I said to Fritz, who occasionally worked on Mrs. Beasley. She adored him. Right now, I certainly couldn't say the same for myself. "I never should have done that."

"Don't worry about it," he replied. "She liked it. I could tell. She's got a good sense of humor."

Well, she certainly didn't fall down on the floor laughing, I thought. I was nervous and disappointed. It was supposed to be a joke.

The next day, I was running from room to room, treating patients during our busiest day, when who should I spot in the waiting room but Mrs. Beasley. Her chipmunk cheeks glowed and her eyes twinkled. What a sweetheart. She beckoned me over, and held up the drawing.

"It took me awhile to figure out what it was," she snorted. "I don't believe it! I love it! I didn't really think you paid that much attention to your patients! This is great! I'm going to show all my girlfriends at bridge today." She got the giggles so hard that tears began to form at the corners of her eyes.

She gave my shoulder a squeeze and danced out the door.

Some patients leave their marks on doctors' souls. Some leave their marks on doctors' egos. Some leave their marks by suing. Or sending thank you notes. Mrs. Beasley left her mark in a more literal way. Hers was the mark of a true aristocrat.

CHAPTER 43

"Gone–glimmering through the dream of things that were."

Lord Byron

I met Andrew in the heat of the summer, when the azaleas were exploding with color and lawns were just starting to turn brown. He had a magnetic personality—the room was filled with people, but something about him drew me to his side, and, before we'd chatted for even five minutes, I felt like we were old buddies.

Andrew was tall and muscular. At about 6'2", he weighed 185 pounds and looked like he spent a lot of time at the gym. His skin was a healthy shade of mahogany, and I noticed a diamond stud in his right earlobe. But when I shook his hand, it was cool and clammy, and when he rose to greet me, it took him several seconds to walk just a couple of feet to where I was standing. It seemed like his ankles were swollen. Something about his eyes, their piercing quality, the way they stared, made me feel very sad, and sent a chill down my spine.

So this is AIDS, I thought.

I'd shown up at the little meeting room to give a talk on chiropractic to a group of AIDS patients. I'd heard about a local AIDS organization, and when I'd discovered that only two medical doctors out of the hundreds who were practicing locally would see AIDS patients, I decided to throw my hat in the ring. Only two doctors would treat these people? I was shocked. And disgusted. Clearly, someone needed to be educated.

I knew that I risked losing a few patients if they were to find out that I treated AIDS victims. People would run the other way, thinking they'd catch it from a sneeze. Chiropractors don't draw blood, perform surgery, or use sharp instruments such as those used in dental work, so the risk was negligible. Even so, others believed that those who had AIDS were vile and deserving of suffering, and that no one should help alleviate their misery.

I had no way of knowing then how important Andrew would be to me or to my practice. All I knew was that he seemed like a nice guy and I thought that I could help him. Later, I would meet many AIDS patients in my practice, but the one who truly broke my heart was the four-year-old hemophiliac girl whose muscles were atrophying to the point where she could hardly walk. She was in a lot of pain. With my adjustments and hot packs, I finally got her to sleep through the night. Her mother was relieved; after two adjustments, her daughter was no longer waking up in tears several times a night. To top it off, they were broke. There was just no way I could charge for those treatments.

During my AIDS lecture the evening I met Andrew, I explained that chiropractic philosophy recognizes the need for drugs to kill pain or to help wipe out bacterial infections, but that, as a day-to-day crutch, drugs were not the answer. Drugs do not cure disease—your body cures disease. Drugs merely give your body an added boost when it needs it.

I told the audience that while no one had yet found a cure for AIDS, chiropractic spinal adjustments could help boost their immune systems and possibly help prevent colds and flu, which could be devastating to AIDS patients. But because the whole premise of AIDS is that your immune system is shot, chiropractic cannot cure it. I told them that chiropractic adjustments could help relieve joint pain and swelling that was typical of the disease. It was this point that the audience members seemed most interested in. Most were on codeine and a variety of painkillers and hated spending so much of their time in a daze, unable to hold down jobs or even talk on the phone.

Andrew was my first adult AIDS patient. I helped bring down the swelling in his ankles, and I spoke to him at length about diet and exercise. Although he didn't yet exhibit the emaciated, frail aura that I would learn to recognize instantly as that of an AIDS patient, he was certainly in no shape to take up running or pole vaulting. I suggested stretches at his bedside every morning and a brisk walk as far as he could go comfortably.

One day, when Andrew came in for his weekly visit, he brought in a friend who was so thin that he could barely walk. His breathing was labored and raspy. His ankles were grossly swollen. His movements were uncoordinated. His speech was slurred.

"Can you help him?" begged Andrew. "He's in so much pain and he's on so many drugs. He doesn't get a good night's sleep, but he's never fully awake, either."

Before I could respond, Andrew's friend dove for the wastebasket and began to vomit. His body shuddered with every retch, and his rib cage protruded through his flimsy T-shirt. At last, he sat on the edge of the treatment table and hung his head, exhausted.

"I'm sorry," I said.

"No, I'm sorry," his friend gasped. "I'll disinfect the wastebasket in the men's room. Do you have anything I could use? Lysol? Bleach?"

Even at death's door, this man was following prescribed societal etiquette. I was impressed. But then, it was more than etiquette—although AIDS is spread by a very slow, weak virus, and no one has yet proven that it can be spread by saliva, no one knows enough about it to be convinced that something like stomach acid can't spread it. Andrew's friend was not only making sure a loaded gun wasn't pointing at me, he was taking out the clip.

Andrew missed his next visit. I wondered if he'd forgotten, if he was ill or if he'd given up on chiropractic. I wondered how his friend was feeling. I hadn't even examined his friend, much less adjusted him. He was too exhausted to make it through the exam. He just wanted to go home and lie down.

That afternoon, I got a personal call from Andrew.

"Randy died this morning," he said. "God, I miss him already. It hurts so much." He sobbed into the phone.

"I'm sorry," I said. "But I'm glad that I got to meet him before he died, Andrew."

That seemed to be just what Andrew needed to hear. He cleared his throat and took a deep breath, and asked if he could reschedule his appointment. I connected him with the front desk.

But when Andrew came in, he was already beginning to show signs of wear. Dark shadows swam beneath his eyes. His mahogany skin was nearly gray. His ankles were swollen again. He was running a fever.

I adjusted his neck because he'd been complaining that his head felt "full." He couldn't pinpoint the location, and couldn't describe the feeling any better than that. I assumed that it was due to the disease and all the drugs he was on. The report sent from his medical doctor listed them: Sinequan, Leukovorin, Mellaril, Naprosin, Retrovir, Codeine and AZT.

He said that the neck adjustments helped him sleep at night and relieved the pain, and I was pleased. Some days when he came in, he couldn't even turn his head sideways. The adjustments gave him a lot more neck mobility. Anything I could do to help would be worth it.

As the weeks went by, Andrew referred more and more AIDS acquaintances. I built up a booming AIDS practice without ever having intended to. Because of my speaking engagements and networking, more and more M.D.s began to treat AIDS patients, as well. Things were looking up.

The only problem was that no one had found a cure. The situation was improving only in that more AIDS patients were seeking help and more were receiving humane treatment to ease their pain until they died. It wasn't long until I realized that Andrew wouldn't be my patient for much longer.

"I'm so exhausted," he complained. "I can't even walk up the stairs to my apartment without stopping for breath every few steps. I've lost so much weight, but I feel like I weigh a ton." His skin was ashen. His hair was dry and brittle. His lips were parched and blistered.

Andrew was now down to 135 lbs. and looking worse every day.

"You know I was discharged from the Navy, don't you?" he asked. Frankly, it hadn't entered my mind, but since he mentioned it, I assumed that it was inevitable.

"I hate their doctors. They wouldn't know compassion if you threw it in their faces. All they want to do is get you to die so they can get rid of you. We're all just an embarrassment to the Navy.

"It's hell knowing that you're going to die," he said, looking up at me, his eyes sunken and pained. "But what's worse is that nobody wants to be with you. The Navy hates me. People I thought were friends have all deserted me. The rest of my friends are dying. Do you know how it feels to have your best friend die? I'm only thirty years old. I'm not ready yet. I have no one. And I can't just say 'screw it' and go for a walk or wander through the mall, because it takes too much energy to go. All I can do is sit in the kitchen and stare out the window or lie in bed and watch TV and feel sorry for myself."

Two weeks later, Andrew got so weak that he quit sleeping upstairs in his bedroom. The stairs were just too much for him. And since he didn't have the energy to drag the mattress down the stairs, he slept on the wooden living room floor with a blanket and pillow.

His weight was now 100 lbs.

When Andrew grew too feeble to come into the clinic, I made house calls. I made him get up and walk out into the hallway, get the mail and the paper. I adjusted his neck, his lower spine, his ankles, his wrists. All his joints were jammed and painful. He was filled with arthritis. His lymph nodes were so swollen on his neck that you could see the bulges from across the room. He'd been on AZT for weeks. I treated him for free.

Eventually, Andrew began to see double and had constant dizzy spells. Even when he was flat on his back, he felt like he was falling and spinning. One of his medical doctors had him tested, and Andrew's I.Q. had fallen by several points. He began to suffer from dementia.

His walls were covered with paintings that he had done before he'd become so weak. They were colorful and abstract and representational. One illustrated a nightmare. It was filled with fangs and spikes. Several looked like rectums. A painting next to the doorway showed a naked, skeletal man hitchhiking along a deserted stretch of highway, utterly alone. I'd always been taught to appreciate art, but

Andrew's art was too far removed from my personal experience for me to appreciate it. But wasn't that true of AIDS, as well?

Andrew began repeating conversations over and over. I found myself listening to a litany of pain and loneliness and, although I could comprehend Andrew's plight intellectually, I could not empathize. Since no one else was coming to Andrew's apartment and couldn't see his artwork, and he wanted desperately to communicate what he was going through, I suggested that he write it down. "Write an essay," I told him. "Write a poem. The only way you can communicate the horror of something as compelling as AIDS is to create some form of art. You've already done it with your paintings. What about poetry? Try a poem."

He tried his best to smile despite the cracked fever blisters on his lips. He reached out a hand and shook mine feebly. "Thanks Dr. J. You'll be the first to see it."

He was true to his word. The result of his work was a poem he called "Trouble in Paradise." I never saw him again in the clinic. Andrew worked on the poem the next week during his stay in the hospital. I visited him and watched him working on it. The phrases came slowly, painfully. His wrists were locked, his joints swollen, filled with arthritis. His writing was nearly illegible. He died two days later.

At his funeral, I gulped hard when a Catholic priest read the poem aloud. I thought that I'd been able to appreciate the verses on paper, but that priest brought the poem alive with his inflections and intonations. The church was packed with all of Andrew's friends. He would have been pleased. He had complained of being alone, but I discovered that what he meant was not that he had no friends, but that he was alone in his suffering. The packed pews attested to the fact that Andrew had not lost his friends at all.

The priest's voice echoed off the walls:

> Come One, Come All, and Listen Well: Have you heard the news? There's Trouble in Paradise. Men, women, and children are dropping like flies all over the land as if they are being exterminated.
>
> You know, this has been going on too long. We must pitch in, every positive way to conquer this deadly and cruel heartbreaking disease.
>
> Have you heard the news? Yes, there is Trouble in Paradise! Humanity frightened and in panic. . .even though love and caring is among us. Jesse Jackson says to "Keep hope alive," and that "We are all somebody and we must keep the dream alive," and that "We are not alone." This gives me comfort and "Rocks my soul in the bosom of Abraham."

By now I'm sure you've all heard the news. Yes. . .There is Trouble in Paradise. It has robbed my body of health, brought in confusion and despair, and it has killed more than I wish to share. It is killing me. . .and many more.

It has made an impact on my faith in God so real that, that in itself, somehow gives me the wonderful opportunity to appreciate the old Negro spiritual, "This little light of mine—I'm going to let it shine. . ." everywhere I go. In my house, in the doctor's office, the hospital, in my community, Yes! my light shall shine, not just for me but for all humanity!

Have you heard the news? Yes, there's Trouble in Paradise! Pass the word, inform all who will listen and take heed that ALL life is precious. Yes, too precious to turn our backs on: The trees, the birds, green grass, even the radiant sunshine; The wetness of the rain, and the powerful life-giving soil, water and air; The entire grace of creation!

I'm sure you've heard the news. . .There's Trouble in Paradise. The Rev. Martin Luther King Jr. coined the phrase, "We shall overcome," which is known all over God's land and also reminds us that longevity has its place.

The surgeon general of the United States, C. Everett Koop, has informed us that "America and the world is experiencing an epidemic," and the only way we can conquer it is to keep trying to find a cure. Some say it's nowhere in sight. Well, I say to what little faith you have, all problems have answers.

To the God of understanding, give praise, thanksgiving and believe. Ask for mercy. Believe in your heart that we can pitch in to comfort, respect all, and share a smile. Reach out and touch men, women and our precious future—children. Remember through the Almighty and our determinant we shall stop the tears of mothers, fathers, sisters and brothers of all afflicted. Joy shall appear all over God's land and we shall be free of this awful deadly disease. Faith in mankind and the Almighty God shall give us the research money; the love and caring and yes, the sweet determination to overcome. Oh to sing, how we got over, and rid the societies of the world of this awful and menacing affliction. Then we shall stand together giving praise to God. We will bind together and shed tears of joy, and never forget that we can ALL help in positive ways to keep hope alive. When it's over, we shall smell the fragrance of the rose, hear the song of birds, feel the mist of the morning and not fear the darkness of night.

Now that you know the news, never forget the Trouble in Paradise: AIDS—Acquired Immune Deficiency Syndrome.

Hopefully, soon, very soon, we can spread the news like wild fire. . ."We have found a cure!"

Remember. . .before you turn your back; before you hang your head in shame; before you lose a friend; before you fall on your knees; AIDS can happen to you. May God forbid!

When it's all over, we will have maintained our sense of self respect, integrity, dignity, and pride in being a part of humanity.

My friends, just before the darkness and the light of eternity closes in, put your arms around me and tell me that you love me.

CHAPTER 44

"Lord Ronald said nothing; he flung himself from the room, flung himself upon his horse and rode madly off in all directions."

Stephen Leacock

There are times when being the only doctor in a busy clinic is the perfect ego trip. You are in total control. The patients expect to be seen only by you. There are no philosophical arguments between you and your colleagues. You handle all the finances. All is peaceful.

And then there are days when you are so busy, you walk into walls. When you feel like Alice, through the looking glass, in a world unreal and altogether unfair. You don't have time to catch your breath, stop for lunch, run to the bathroom. Those are the days when another doctor is a gift from heaven.

We were booked solid. And Murphy's Law was in effect. On top of the scheduled patients, we got walk-ins: patients who just happened to be passing by and decided they wanted a treatment. Or patients who'd been in accidents and decided to see us instead of going for a ride in an ambulance to spend four hours in the emergency room only to be sent home with instructions to use a heating pad and oh—don't forget the bill for $400.

I walked in the door, expecting to greet Fritz with a cup of coffee, relax at my desk, plan out my day, and do a little paperwork. But, to my surprise, there were already two patients in the reception area: walk-ins. Walk-ins always take a little longer, because I have to do a history and a complete exam.

By 9:00 A.M., I was already running behind. Every single room was full, and the reception area was overflowing. "How do you do it?" Fritz asked. Fritz Dillard had a tendency to move very, very slowly. He sat and chatted with each patient as if he were enjoying a lunch date. His conversations were irrelevant in regard to the patients' reasons for being there. It irked me to hear him chatting convivially behind a closed exam door when there were a half-dozen patients in the reception area and I was singlehandedly caring for four more. I half expected to hear the "Pssffft" of a beer can being popped open.

I was trying to train Dillard to ask pertinent questions that made it sound like he was chatting with the patient, but which actually aided in his diagnosis. For example, one of my Midwestern patients was having pains down his left arm, shortness of breath, and dizzy spells. I asked him what he'd done that morning. Watched TV? Played with his grandchildren? The gray-haired fellow chuckled and said that his grandchildren were in school, so he'd taken advantage of the free time to shovel the walk. About two inches of snow had fallen that morning. Come to think of it, that's when the pain in his arm began. . .

Voilà! He was sent to the hospital in an ambulance and my clues all added up correctly: he was having a heart attack.

I outlined a sample script for Dr. Dillard that he could use when questioning patients who'd been in car accidents. "Ask them how fast they were going, and what direction the other car was coming from," I suggested. "You need to determine the angle that the patient was hit so you can decide if it's a simple case of whiplash or something more complicated. Ask detailed questions. It's easy. People always want to talk about their car accidents."

That day, I sat in with Dr. Dillard as he questioned one of his first car-accident patients. He told me that he'd understood the reason for asking questions and knew that they would help him in making a diagnosis.

"So, I heard you were in a car accident, Patty," he said. "What happened?"

"I don't know," she said, "it all happened so fast."

Fritz looked baffled and disappointed, but I was undaunted. Aha, I thought, this is the perfect opportunity to ask specific questions and figure out exactly what happened. Sometimes I even had a patient draw me a map. Such specifics also helped later if the patient decided to seek legal counsel.

I'd been an expert witness in a case where a woman rear-ended a car that had stopped at a green light because a fire engine went roaring through the intersection with no warning. After the woman slammed into the car in front of her, she was rear-ended from behind. To add insult to injury, her seat collapsed and sent her catapulting into the back seat, where her head hit the back seat cushion and her neck jammed. She distinctly remembered hearing a "crunch." I wasn't able to sit in on the entire trial, of course, but I found out later that the woman won her case against the city and against the auto manufacturer for a defective seat. My only role in the case was to report her injuries to the jury.

Dr. Dillard had paused long enough and his questions were ready to burst out, unrestrained. He'd determine the exact angle that Patty's car was struck. He'd know exactly how much force was exerted. He'd know if she was thrown against her seat belt and the steering wheel, or whether her legs had flown up, smashing her shins against the dashboard.

He took a deep breath, and with a peculiar note of confidence, he asked, "What color was the car that hit you?"

I groaned and, catching myself, tried to make it sound like I was clearing my throat. "Were you stopped at an intersection?" I offered.

Even so, I wished that Fritz were there to help me out on another day. I could whine about his antics as much as I wanted, but the simple fact was, he helped me out immensely. Most patients were on planned treatment programs that included therapy, and the procedure was simple and fast. But I had no time for wishing. I had a bursitis in Room 2, a disc in Room 3, a whiplash in Room 4, arthritis in Room 5, and a new patient with carpal tunnel syndrome in the exam room.

"How do you do it?" Dillard's question rang in my ears. How? It had nothing to do with school. Nothing to do with knowing which patients would take more time than others. And everything to do with the years I'd spent as a waiter at Steak and Ale.

Being a good waiter means that you have to have an innate sense of timing and a knack for detecting a variety of personalities.

Being a good waiter means that you have to plan out every minute and every inch of floor space. You know exactly how the tables are lined up, which ones were seated first and which ones are ready to leave. That means that when you bring out the desserts for the last two tables, you pick up the dirty plates from the first table on your way back. When you serve the middle table, you also bring out the waters for table next to it, and the drinks for table beyond that.

A lousy waiter will take the order for the middle table and bring it back to the kitchen without so much as a backward glance at any of the other tables. Then, ignoring that food in the kitchen that's up for the table at the end, he'll skip to the next table and ask them if they'd like water. He does all this in plain view of all the tables, infuriating them, because they can see that his hands are almost always empty, he's waiting on everyone except for them, and they're getting hungry and tired.

I memorized the patients in every treatment room. I knew that since the new patient in the exam room would take up most of my physical time, I had to treat all the other patients in some form, leave them waiting for a few moments, then come back to them. Luckily for my schedule, most of their injuries today required that they be put on therapy. To ensure that I'd be back promptly to remove the therapies, I memorized the times for their therapies—anywhere from seven to twenty minutes. In between the therapies, I would take a new patient's history, then give him instructions to don a dressing gown. During that time, I'd remove the hot and cold packs from the patient in another room, adjust that patient, and send him on his way.

Then I'd return to the new patient, do the exam, and determine whether he needed an x-ray. I'd instruct him to get dressed, then go back to one of the interferential patients, take him off therapy and adjust him. Then I'd put the new patient in one of treatment rooms that had just opened up and put him on ice and heat for pain only, since I hadn't completed my diagnosis yet.

By that time, another half-dozen patients had been placed in treatment rooms during different intervals and I was ready to begin the cycle all over again.

Sometimes, I felt like my activities would look great in fast motion on black and white film, paired with Keystone Cops music. Those are the days when I look at the clock and wonder if it's broken when the big hand is on the 7 and the little hand is on the 8. I've been here for twelve hours? What about lunch? Dinner? Uh-oh—I forgot to call my wife.

At least, being a waiter offered the reward of a snack at the end of the evening and some fellow waiters and waitresses to share it with. Party time! Being a doctor offered the reward of knowing I'd gotten several dozen people out of pain, while my clinic looked like it had been used as a bomb shelter.

CHAPTER 45

"It's no longer a question of staying healthy. It's a question of finding a sickness that you like."

Jackie Mason

The peaceful white glow of individual colonial candle lights in the windows of cozy homes up and down the block lent a greeting-card atmosphere to the neighborhood. The pungent odor of burning wood tickled my nostrils as I stepped out the front door. What was it about the holidays that always made me feel like humming? I pulled the door shut behind me, preparing to take a ride over to Jack and Sandy's house for Christmas Eve festivities. Terry was already there with the baby, helping with last-minute preparations. But it wasn't meant to be. My pager went off. Who could it possibly be? A patient wishing me Merry Christmas? An overachiever who fell off the ladder while decorating the tree?

When I heard Dan's voice on the answering machine, I knew it was something important. He wouldn't call me on a holiday unless it was urgent. I returned the call.

"Hey, I'm really sorry about bothering you on Christmas Eve, but I was wrestling with my son on the living room floor and I think I really hurt him. I twisted his neck. He's been crying for over an hour now. Can we come in?"

"Sure." I hopped in the car and met them at the clinic. Dan was right: his son was really messed up. Dave had twisted his shoulder and messed up his neck.

After examining Dave's neck, I iced him, gave him five minutes of muscle relaxation techniques, then set about adjusting him. At twelve years old, he was very easy to adjust, and every single vertebra moved precisely as it should after I'd finished. The pain ceased immediately. He had a rib out of place, too, and when I adjusted that, the "pop" it made could be heard across the room.

Dave was standing and stretching blissfully and I told him to take it easy. He was fascinated with all the equipment. He seemed not to mind the pain at all—it was almost worth the trip to my office just for the adventure of it all.

Dave was like a new person. I didn't even schedule him for another appointment. I suggested a maintenance plan every few months, and Dave and his dad took a few pamphlets to show the rest of the family. I loved adjusting kids—they healed so fast!

"Dan, pick on someone your own size next time," I said.

"Yeah, I should have known better," he said.

"Why don't you buy Dave karate lessons for Christmas?" I suggested. "Then in a few months, when you come in all bruised and beaten, I can tell Dave to pick on someone his own size!"

They both laughed and wished me a Merry Christmas—and I still made it to Jack and Sandy's house in time to open all the kids' gifts.

Mandy showed up at the clinic the Monday after New Year's with a kink in her toe. That's right—her toe. She limped across the floor and down the hall, gingerly lifting her toes and putting most of the pressure on her heel.

I could clearly see that the muscle was spasmed out, and the toe, the one right next to the big toe, was out of joint. Mandy had been in once before when she hurt her lower back, but I hadn't seen her for several months. She chatted a bit, brought me up to date on things that had happened lately.

I pulled on the toe quickly, giving it a hard jerk, and immediately heard a "pop." Mandy gasped. She reached down and rubbed the area. "Look," she said, "it's normal! How did you do that so fast?"

"It only took me eight years of school and thousands of toes," I quipped.

She laughed. Then she blushed furiously and looked away. "I can't believe I did that to my toe. It was really stupid," she said.

I'd never seen anyone blush that hard, and suddenly she piqued my curiosity. I knew that she had a cat and a dog, and I pictured her down on all fours, roughhousing with them.

"You sound embarrassed about your toe," I replied.

She looked up at me imploringly. Then, steeling herself, she braced her shoulders, and with all the dignity she could muster, said, "I was having sex. And that's all I'm going to tell you."

It struck me funny that she felt obligated to tell me; I hadn't even asked. I caught myself grinning, and slapped a serious expression on my face. "Hmmm," I said, running a forefinger across my chin, as though contemplating the matter. "That's not altogether uncommon. You'd be surprised at how many people do that."

"They do?" she gasped. "I had no idea. That makes me feel better."

What a hero, I thought, although I now wondered if she'd tell me exactly what she'd been doing during sex at the time she spasmed out her toe.

"Dr. Joseph, D-1," Clara said.

Oh, well. I guess I'd just never know.

Sam strode into the office like a lumberjack. A former champion bodybuilder, he practically lived at the gym. That is, when he wasn't hanging out at the pizza parlor, snarfing pepperonis and guzzling beer.

"I messed up my shoulder," he said.

"Let me take a look at it," I replied. He pulled off his T-shirt with a great deal of effort. I would have helped him with it, but I knew from seeing him at the gym that he was too macho to allow me. He must have been in excruciating pain to have even considered coming to the clinic.

I motioned out his shoulder and he winced. His biceps bulged. His neck, expanded and corded like rope, was red and hot to the touch. His shoulder was puffed out, ripe like a melon.

"Rotary cuff problem," I said. "I'm going to do some trigger point work, then some stretching, then an adjustment."

"Fine."

I dug my fingers into the affected area and it wasn't long before I started to feel fatigued. I switched fingers, then began using my thumb. I'd worked on a lot of people before, but Sam was a tough one. His muscles were huge and had once been perfectly developed—a doctor's dream to examine because you could see the individual muscle fibers peeking through the skin. But now, his muscles were turning to mush and all I could feel was layers of fat. He was hell to palpate.

I could see that my efforts were having an effect. Sam was gritting his teeth from the pain, and the triggers were reduced already. I began to stretch him. Again, he grimaced, and I coaxed him to relax his shoulder as much as possible. "You can do it," I said. "Come on, just a couple more seconds." Just like working out at the gym—a little more, you can do it, push, push, breathe, hold it. . .

Finally, I was ready for the adjustment. By the time I'd finished the trigger-point work and the stretching, the area was already much improved, but the adjustment would be the final and most important touch.

The sudden crack from the adjustment startled Sam. He held his breath for a moment while I massaged the area. "How's that?" I said.

He moved the shoulder gingerly. Then he lifted the arm over his head, and dropped it back down. He rotated it. He shrugged his shoulders. He struck a pose, clowning in front of the mirror. "Great, doc! It's perfect!"

He smacked me on the back, and grabbed my shoulder in a friendly embrace on his way out the door. I was happy for him. But I wasn't smiling. He'd nearly dislocated my shoulder! I'd underestimated Sam—he still had a lot of life in those muscles. What a grip! I unbuttoned my shirt and pulled down the collar to see if I'd been bruised. Whew—that was a close one.

But not all patients walked out the door after one treatment and pronounced themselves cured. Some were ecstatic if they were only partially improved, even after several visits. Mark was only eighteen years old, but already he'd lost almost 80 percent of his hearing. He wore hearing aids in both ears, and they were huge. "Aren't these a little outdated?" I asked him.

"Yeah, but they're too expensive to replace."

"Maybe you could get on some kind of a payment plan somewhere," I suggested. "These just really look old."

Mark had been coming in for the past three weeks for neck and ear adjustments. The ear has three tiny bones that can be adjusted, simply by pulling the earlobe down and angled out with a swift motion. But Mark said he thought that the earlobe adjustment was helping his hearing—he'd been able to turn down the volume on his hearing aids since he'd been coming to see me.

Anything was possible. But I think it was more likely that it was the neck adjustments I was doing. After all, that's how D.D. Palmer made chiropractic famous in the first place—restoring someone's hearing with a neck adjustment. The earlobe adjustment works better for patients with ear infections—it helps take the bite out of the pain.

Eventually, Mark bought a new set of hearing aids. They were more compact, much more modern. He was pleased. And more than that, he was thrilled because he'd had his hearing checked and now had only a 50-percent loss. The audiologist was surprised. It was rare to find a patient with such improvement. Most folks with hearing aids had damage to the little hairs inside the ear, and, once destroyed, the hairs can never be replaced. Mark was lucky that part of his problem had been nerve impingement and it had improved.

An audiologist is a handy person when it comes to referrals. I'd referred several car accident patients to an audiologist. I adjusted their necks and gave them traction, but when it became evident that their dizziness was getting worse, I referred them out. The audiologist could determine if they had an inner-ear problem that could be resolved through pressure sensitivity exercises.

Chiropractors see such an array of illnesses that their practices often resemble family practice medical doctors' practices. Aside from hearing problems, rotary cuff manifestations or spasmed toes, we also see arthritis cases, wry neck, headaches and bursitis. Sometimes, there's no problem at all; patients just misinterpret the noises and physical messages their bodies send. One such case caught me off guard and I threw my sensitivity to the wind, not to mention my manners.

Jimmy Sapper was brought into the clinic because his mother was concerned about the fact he cracked his knuckles incessantly.

"It's not good for him," she complained. "He's gotten so bad that I just know he's going to have arthritis by the time he's fourteen." Jimmy was thirteen.

Mrs. Sapper was, in a word, a pain. She picked on every little thing that Jimmy did, and, from everything I could see, he appeared normal. He was just an adolescent. . .If anyone going through adolescence could be considered normal.

He was driving his mother up the wall, and evidently I had been chosen as the intermediary. "There's nothing wrong with knuckle-cracking, Mrs. Sapper," I said. Her eyebrows shot up.

"The sound you're hearing is carbon dioxide being released between the joints. It's perfectly normal." As I spoke, I motioned out all of Jimmy's fingers, showing him how each joint could move in six different directions. He was fascinated, and clearly pleased that I'd let him off the hook.

But not so fast. "I'm paying good money to have you tell me that Jimmy isn't hurting himself?" ranted Mrs. Sapper. "Why, I've never heard such a thing. I felt sure you'd tell me he was going to cut off all the circulation and I'd just watch gangrene set in and then where would we be?" Her lips, pencil thin, twitched, and she peered over the tops of her glasses with beady gray eyes.

"It's simply the sound of air being released," I repeated. I then picked up Mrs. Sapper's right hand and began to motion out the joints. I found a jammed joint and adjusted it. It made a popping sound. She gasped and Jimmy snickered.

"You may want to crack your knuckles every now and then yourself, Mrs. Sapper," I said. "Keep those joints moving.The only problem is," I paused for effect, clasping the fingers of both my hands together in a palms up fashion, preparing to crack all ten at once, "that it's *obnoxious.* " I cracked the whole lot, sending Mrs. Sapper into a tizzy and Jimmy into a snit of laughter.

"Anything else?" I asked, opening the door. Mrs. Sapper stared at me, mute. "Fine. Oh, and there's no charge for the visit."

I strode down the hallway, Mrs. Sapper's scowl the last thing I saw as I turned to leave.

CHAPTER 46

"Pleasure is oft a visitant; but pain clings cruelly to us."

John Keats, *Endymion*

Luke made a good living as a plumber, but lately he'd been taking off so much time from work because of his back that he'd be lucky if he could make a living at all.

Luke was referred to me by a mutual friend. When he came in, he could hardly walk. He held his body in an unnaturally stiff position and limped across the floor.

"When did this happen?" I asked.

"Oh, a couple weeks ago. I was twisting underneath this lady's sink to install a garbage disposal and I guess I just twisted the wrong way. I barely made it through the job, and making it out the door was really rough."

"Do you do a lot of twisting like that?" I asked.

"You kiddin'? I've been underneath people's crawlspaces, in their attics, inside their bathtubs and showers. I go everywhere. Even in the yard. Sometimes tree roots grow like crazy and work their way into pipes and clog the hell out of 'em. I don't know why people think that plumbers have it so easy."

He was in so much pain that sweat trickled down his forehead and clumps of stringy hair stuck to his face. When he spoke, his sentences were chopped into fragments, punctuated by shallow breaths.

"When do you notice the pain the most?" I asked.

"When I sneeze!" he said, cracking a smile for the first time.

"Okay," I said, "let's try some tests."

I ran him through a series of chiropractic and orthopedic tests and nearly every movement caused him to cry out in pain. One of the most painful involved the least amount of movement: all he had to do was stand up straight, then drop his chin to his chest.

He also had pain radiating down his leg, and any walking aggravated it. Everything pointed to a herniated disc, but I always treat conservatively before sending out for an MRI. This appeared to be something that I could treat with adjustments, traction and ice packs.

"I'll tell you what, Luke. I'm going to treat you for two weeks. If your problem improves, we'll continue with the treatment. If it gets worse, I'm going to send you out for an MRI."

"What's an MRI?"

"Magnetic Resonance Imaging," I said. "It's safer than x-rays and it provides a great picture. But you have to take off time from work to do it, and it's expensive. So let's wait a couple weeks and see how you do."

He agreed. We began the treatment program and within two days Luke was so much better that I knew that my working diagnosis was correct. He had no more pain radiating down his leg, and he could bend and twist just like he used to.

Luke felt so good, as a matter of fact, that he quit coming in altogether and proceeded to install another garbage disposal. He re-injured himself and was brought directly to my office by his wife. It took three of my staff members to carry him into the clinic.

I re-examined him. The exam showed that he was much worse than he was during the original exam. I x-rayed him. I iced the area, then adjusted his lower spine. I also ran electrotherapy because the muscles around the area had spasmed out.

"Luke," I said, "I'm going to take you off work for the rest of the week." He started to object but I kept on talking. "I want you to ice the area several times a day, and I don't want you installing any more garbage disposals until you are totally healed. When I get you out of pain, that doesn't mean you are totally healed and that you stop coming in. It simply means that you're out of pain. You've seen the x-rays. We have to go beyond that and take care of the problem. After you're healed, you're going to start on an exercise program. First, it will just involve stretches. Later, I want you to build up your abdominals."

I patted his ample belly. "Too much fat here messes up your weight distribution and puts pressure on your spine." His face reddened. "If you lose this extra weight and keep up with your stretches, you should be able to change fifty garbage disposals a day."

He sighed and shook his head. He was miserable. But the good part was that I knew I could help him.

After two weeks of adjustments and therapy, his sciatica again disappeared and he was able to get dressed in the morning without help. Mainly, that meant that his wife didn't have to help him put on his socks because until this point, he hadn't been able to bend over to do it.

"We've got you out of pain," I warned, "but you're not all better.

You've still got a disc problem and muscle tension." He was face down on a treatment table so I emphasized the point by digging my thumb into his lower spine. He winced.

"Keep up the good work, Luke. You're doing great."

Luke only had one minor setback. He was bringing in a few bags of groceries and started experiencing lower back pain. "I think my wife thought I'd made it up because I didn't want to bring in the rest of the groceries," he laughed, "but boy, did that sucker hurt! I was in bed for the rest of the day!"

"Did you remember to put pillows under your knees to take pressure off your back?" I reminded him.

"Yeah, yeah," he said. "I remembered."

Within six weeks after Luke's re-injury, he was back at work, installing garbage disposals. He was as happy as a clam.

"I thought I was going to end up having surgery," he confessed. "I sure was scared for a while."

I hadn't told him that after an MRI, surgery is often the next step. He'd figured it out by himself. "The majority of lower back surgeries fail," I said. "Did you know that?"

He looked shocked. "No. Now I'm really glad I didn't have surgery."

"If your disc had been fully sequestered—that is, if a fragment had totally separated from the rest of the disc—you wouldn't have had a choice," I said. "You were very lucky that your injury wasn't that severe. You know, doctors have something we call the 80-10-10 rule. Eighty percent of the patients who walk through the front door can be helped. Ten percent must be referred out. And 10 percent cannot be helped at all. Those are the patients who keep doctors awake at night. For both of our sakes, I'm glad you're not in that 10 percent."

The next day, Joe Grass came in. He'd been in before a couple of times. Joe was a construction worker and spent his days sweating in the hot sun, lugging around equipment and running a jackhammer. He always reeked of cigarette smoke, and I could tell by his gut that he drank a lot of beer.

I asked him what brand he drank. "You're not going to recommend that lite stuff, are you? That stuff is for sissies. You stick to advice about my back, doc, and I'll get my bartender to stick to advice about my beer."

Joe had tattoos on both arms. His conversation was smattered with four-letter words. His muddy footprints followed us to room 3.

"What seems to be the problem?" I asked.

"I got this weird pain in my calves," he said, rubbing them. "I guess it's from standing all day. And every now and then my lower back tightens up, but it ain't too bad."

I brought in Dr. Dillard and explained to him what was going on.

Any time there was something new and unusual, I liked to bring him in not only to educate him, but in case he came up with an idea.

But Dillard hadn't a clue. So after the exam and x-ray, I adjusted Joe's lower spine and put him on interferential current. I attached one of the pads to the area just to the right of his lower spine, and the other two pads I placed on his calf.

After three days, there was absolutely no change in Joe's condition. "How do you feel, Joe?" I asked.

"The same," he said. "My calves are killin' me, and my lower back is still stiff."

"I'm going to send you out for an MRI, Joe," I said. "I'd like to rule out a sequestered disc."

The MRIs came back showing a fully sequestered disc. Joe was sent to a surgeon. Dr. Dillard was flabbergasted. "What about all the pain?" he fairly shouted. "That guy hardly complained at all. We have patients who complain like they're going to die, and it's just a pulled muscle. How did you know?"

"Do you know what really did it for me? It wasn't any of the symptoms; it was the fact that Joe actually complained. I mean, he's been in here for all sorts of things, and he really keeps his mouth shut. He broke a toe awhile back during a hot shot back-yard football game, and the only reason he came in was because his girlfriend made him. You could crush a cigarette out in Joe's hand and he wouldn't even flinch.

"Which, by the way, reminds me of a theory I heard from a guy at the American Back Society. He said that smoking is related to degenerative disc disease and sequestered discs. Joe smokes, you know. When I heard that theory, I went through all my patient files and, sure enough, all my sequestered discs belonged to smokers."

"Whaddaya know," said Dillard.

A week later, I saw a new patient for exactly the same thing Luke, the plumber, had—a bulging disc. She was only twenty-eight years old and had just had a baby.

"What happened, Lois?" I asked.

"I never did get back into shape after having the baby," she said, "and I knew that I should really be doing some situps to strengthen my abdominals, but I just never had the time. Every bit of free time I used to clean the house, write letters or sleep.

"Anyway, I was leaning over the crib to pick up the baby, and I heard this 'pop' and thought I'd die. It felt like someone stabbed me. Then, this pain started racing down my leg and I couldn't even walk. It was awful."

"Did you pick up the baby like this?" I asked, demonstrating the typical way that people bend over to pick up babies and small objects from the floor or a short table. I kept my knees straight and stretched my calf muscles until they threatened to snap.

"Yes," she replied. "Just like that."

"Don't ever do that again," I chastised her. "Always, always, always bend your knees."

She went through a treatment program almost identical to Luke's. And then she came in one day and the minute I saw her, I knew that she'd re-injured herself. Her skin was pallid and her eyes were sunken.

"What happened?" I asked.

"I was doing so well, Dr. Joseph, and then this happened. I was driving along, and the baby started to fuss in the back seat. I reached around to give her a bottle, and it was like I got stuck in position. Gawd, it hurt! I just twisted the wrong way. I'm lucky I didn't run off the road."

My pulse began to quicken as I imagined this twenty-eight-year-old new mother undergoing disc surgery as her anxious and nervous husband took care of the baby for a month.

I carefully conducted the customary series of chiropractic and orthopedic tests, and to my surprise they all came out negative! "Lie face down on the table, Lois," I said.

Before I even touched her, I could see what the problem was. The entire right side of her back right next to the spine was raised, like a snake writhing beneath the skin. Her muscles had spasmed out.

"Give me your hand, Lois," I said. I guided her fingers across the area.

"What is it?" she said. "It's all lumpy."

"You're hypertonic," I said. "Your muscles have spasmed out. We're going to give you lots of therapy and if the hypertonicity has gone down enough by tomorrow, I'll adjust you." I heaved a sigh of relief that it wasn't a disc.

"And Lois," I said, "promise me something. The next time the baby cries when you're driving, pull over and open the back door to give her the bottle, okay?"

"Okay, Dr. J.," she replied. "You know, lots of people warned me that being a mother would be hard on my privacy and hard on my emotions, but no one told me that it would be so hard on my back."

"Motherhood is full of surprises, Lois," I said. "By the way, how did you hear about our office?"

"My plumber told me," she said. "He threw out his back, and he was ready to go back to work in a week. I figured he must have gone to the right place."

I chuckled to myself. A week, eh? So that's where Joe really messed himself up—at Lois' house. Whaddaya know.

CHAPTER 47

"Life is too short to stuff a mushroom."

Storm Jameson

Andrea showed up in the clinic in an awful mood. She barked at the receptionist, bumped into another patient, and plunked herself down on the couch. She grabbed a couple of magazines and flipped through them so fast that she practically ripped out the pages. Her hands trembled and occasionally she'd rub her temples as though she had a headache.

When I brought her into the exam room, I asked her to put on a gown and she rolled her eyes and sighed. "Do I have to? I'm in a hurry to go somewhere and I need to get something to eat and I don't see the point."

"You'll receive a more thorough exam with the gown," I said, "because I can better see your body type, and whether you have any rashes or lesions or bruises. I promise I'll hurry. I'm very busy, too."

When I returned to Andrea, she was seated on the exam table wearing the gown. She held a magazine in her lap, but appeared uninterested in its contents. Her mood had improved to the point that she was laughing and joking. Even so, I could sense an underlying tension.

As I began to examine her, I noticed that her symptoms were contradictory. Her pulse was racing, but her blood pressure was only 102/60. She complained of stress headaches, but she was relaxed to the point of drowsiness. Her hands trembled and she dropped the keys and book I'd given her to test her grasp, but her gait was steady. Occasionally, her speech was slurred, and she'd stare beyond me as though she were off in another world; then suddenly she'd perk up and rattle off statistics and information. I could see that she was intelligent, driven, compulsive and in all other physical respects, normal, except that the curve in her neck was almost nonexistent. I'd have to work on that.

Her weight was a little low for her height—she was 5'4" and weighed 98 lbs.

"Have you lost a lot of weight lately?" I asked.

"No," she replied. "I've always been like this. I eat whatever I want."

"What about your bowel habits?"

"I've got a spastic colon, but other than that, everything is normal."

Hmmm, I thought. Most of my patients with irritable bowel syndrome are high-strung. I made a note of it.

"Have you seen a dentist about your headaches?" I asked.

"Yes," she said. "He told me that most people would die for a bite like mine."

So much for temporal mandibular joint problems, I thought.

"Why?" she asked.

"I just wanted to rule out TMJ," I said, checking the motion. "Are you on the pill?" I asked.

"Yes."

"Have you ever had migraines?"

"Yes, twice this summer. My OB/GYN reduced the dosage on my pills and it helped. He wants to take me off the pill altogether but I'm afraid to. I have screwy periods and it helps regulate them. Besides, I'm not ready to get pregnant."

"I'd really have to agree with your OB/GYN, so think about going off the pill." I noted that she'd been married for seven years and had no children. "I'll show you some things you can do to help you with your cramps. In regard to your neck, I'll set you up for cervical adjustments—that is, neck adjustments—a couple times a week. I want to restore the curve in your neck. That will help relieve your headaches.

"In addition, I'd like you to go out and buy a journal and keep a list of everything you eat for the next two months. That means vitamins, birth control pills, aspirin, candy, and your three meals a day. You have to carry the journal with you because you'll never remember to record it all at the end of the day. You'd be surprised at the things you put in your mouth that you're not even aware of. List everything in columns. Put the date and time on the far left, then the food item in the middle, then on the far right, any symptoms you experience. The symptoms don't have to occur at the same time you eat. Just jot anything down and record the time."

At the end of two months, a distinct pattern emerged. This woman ate everything she could stuff in her mouth. I was amazed that she stayed so slim. She had the metabolism of a hummingbird. Her weight held itself between 98 and 103 lbs.

The neck adjustments helped immensely with the duration and frequency of her stress headaches, but, despite everything, Andrea succumbed to another migraine. It shot her whole weekend. She spent several hours one night throwing up, then several more hours with an ice pack at the base of her skull. Every pain pill she swallowed, she threw up.

Her upturned nose, luminous brown eyes and lush lips gave her a distinctly youthful look, but it wasn't difficult to tell that she was sick. Andrea talked a lot about the stress in her life. It was obvious that her workload and home life were not something she could cope with well. Even so, I couldn't figure out why she was still having migraines. "Are you still on the pill?" I asked.

"Not since last weekend," she said. "After that migraine, I quit." That migraine was actually the best thing that could have happened to Andrea. It was the proverbial straw that broke the camel's back.

One afternoon, she came in around 4 P.M. and, while her mood was pleasant, she was obviously uncomfortable and irritable. She was hiding it well. All except for her trembling hands.

"When was the last time you ate?"

"This morning. I had a bowl of Cocoa Puffs at about 7:30. Oh, and a Coke at 1:00."

Great, I thought. Not only sugar, but caffeine, as well. "Why haven't you eaten since then?"

"I haven't had time."

I asked to see her journal. As I flipped through it, I could see that although she ate everything from here to Mars, it was opportunistic eating—she ate when it was convenient, and when it was inconvenient, she starved. She had no set pattern. In addition to sporadic grazing, she filled the gaps with sugary items—candy, sugar-coated cereal, soda pop. She lived off of Coke and iced tea.

"Have you ever been tested for diabetes?" I asked.

"Yes, several times," she said. "My mother had me tested every couple of years when I was little because I ate so much candy."

Smart mother, I thought. She was on the right track. But just a little off. "Andrea, I think you have a blood sugar problem, but it's not diabetes. It's—"

"Hypoglycemia," she interrupted.

"What made you say that?"

"My mother came up with the idea the other day. I meant to tell you."

Darn! There's nothing worse than having someone's mother steal your diagnosis away from you!

"Is something wrong?" she said.

"Uh, no, I'm glad that we've reached a consensus. You have low blood sugar. You're going to keep the journal going and change your diet. You're going off all sugar. That means no Cheerios, no Frosted Mini Wheats, no Cocoa Puffs, no chocolate, no cream puffs. And no carameled apples."

Her eyes were so wide and her face so pale, I worried that she'd pass out on me right there. Her skin was a medium shade of cocoa, but when her headaches came on, her complexion turned blotchy and she had grayish bags under her eyes. Her black hair, very coarse and naturally wavy, grew stiff and dull. She was a very attractive lady, but anyone could tell by a brief glance that she felt rotten.

"No chocolate?" she said. "How long do I have to do this?"

"Forever," I replied. Little tears began to pool in her eyes.

"Oh, and no caffeine. I noticed in your journal that you drink a lot of Coke and iced tea. You've got to cut that out, too. Also," I added, "no alcohol. Especially red wine."

"All at once?"

"No. We'll start with sugar first. Candy and snacks will be the easiest to cut out because it's easy to keep track of them. You can change two habits in a minimum of twenty-one days. I'll give you thirty days. Replace anything you give up with your favorite fruit, like an apple or a banana. Since you've gone so long without food today, why don't we do a simple blood test just to check your blood-sugar level? Then we can decide whether to do the extended five-hour test to confirm the diagnosis."

She agreed, and, after I called ahead, she ran across the street to the family practice clinic to have blood drawn. She came back a half-hour later with the results. Her blood sugar was so low, I couldn't believe she could walk.

"I guess I have to go in for the long test, huh?" she said. Her hands were shaking so badly, she sat on them.

"No. I think you've been through enough today. Since this test was so conclusive, you can skip more tests and just treat the symptoms with diet. A better diet certainly can't hurt."

After a month, she didn't seem to be improving. "I'm miserable," she complained. "My headaches are a lot better, but I'm so tired all the time. I can't concentrate. When will I see something happening?"

"It takes awhile," I said. "Not only do you have to get all that sugar out of your system, but you have to train your adrenals to produce the correct amount of insulin. What we're going to do now is take you off caffeine."

She sighed.

A month passed. "You're doing great, I said. "According to your journal, you only cheated once this month. Now, I'm going to put you on an exercise program."

"Oh, gawd," she groaned.

"It will help your diet," I pushed. "You've still got a lot of excess adrenaline rushing through your body and it doesn't have anywhere to go. What's happening is that when you eat sugar, your blood sugar level shoots up and your body produces more insulin than it needs. Then the blood sugar comes crashing down, and you get the blues. Some people even get psychotic. It's really sad when little kids have blood sugar problems or food allergies, because when they go berserk, everyone just assumes that they're brats and the kids get punished, when, in reality, they should be put on diets. Anyway, you need to stick to your diet more closely. You've still got too much sugar in it, and you want to avoid that sugar rush."

"Are you kidding? I gave up everything already!"

I opened her journal and pointed to an entry. "Hamburger with ketchup. Ketchup has sugar. Ritz crackers. Lots of sugar. Oriental stir fry. Loaded with sugar."

"You've got to be kidding! There's nothing left to eat! I'll starve!"

"Just learn to read labels more carefully," I coaxed her. "I'll give you a list that will help you recognize different types of sugar on labels at the grocery store. Make your own food so you know what's in it. There are lots of recipe books in health food stores that have sugar-free recipes. They're great."

"I don't have time to cook!" she whined. "I'm too busy; I have to work two jobs!"

"Yes, you do have time to cook," I said. "How much sleep do you get a night? Ten hours? You don't need that much. Once you get your body on track and start exercising, your body will be more efficient and you'll sleep more deeply. You'll find that you'll be able to get by on eight hours with no problem. And how much time did you waste taking naps to get rid of your headaches? Four hours a week? That's where all your lost time is going."

She couldn't help but see my point. She walked out the door shaking her head. But she was a trooper. She showed up in a week, recipe book in tow, smiling. "I've joined the Y," she said. "I'm taking aerobics. I slept through the night without waking up once last night. No nightmares."

"Nightmares? You never told me about nightmares."

"Oh, sorry. They come on whenever I have caffeine or alcohol. Especially coffee drinks. You know, like Kahlua coffee or Irish coffee with lots of whipped cream. And a straw. . .And chocolate shavings." She sighed and gazed out the window. I could see that she was mentally savoring the aroma.

"Actually, I didn't figure that out. My mother did."

"Oh," I said.

When her two months were up, I cut her visits down to once a month. While the curve in her neck was nearly restored, I was still adjusting her neck to take care of any nerve interference and open up the blood flow, and everything else was going well.

After six months, she was like a new person. Her moodiness had evaporated. She was sleeping like a baby. She loved aerobics. And she'd gone hunting at the grocery store and discovered caffeine-free tea, Grape Nuts and Shredded Wheat. She'd even forced herself to watch the clock and eat at prescribed times, even when she thought she wasn't hungry or was certain she was too busy. She'd commented on several occasions that better health had enabled her to more easily deal with the stress in her life. She said she was more clearheaded and better able to make decisions, thereby avoiding stressful situations altogether. The gray circles had disappeared from beneath her eyes.

"You're doing great, Andrea. I'm really impressed. Keep your journal for a year." She looked pleased. "How's your spastic colon?" I felt that it was time to move on to the rest of her symptoms. "You know, Andrea—"

"I'm trying to avoid stressful situations and stay away from greasy, fried foods," she said.

"How did you know that?" I asked.

"My mother told me."

"Oh." I should have known. "Your mother isn't a doctor, is she, Andrea?"

"Oh, no," Andrea laughed. "She just thinks she is!"

"What does she do for a living?" I inquired.

"She owns a candy store. Why?"

"Never mind," I said. "Never mind."

CHAPTER 48

"The only thing that saves us from the bureaucracy is its inefficiency."

Eugene McCarthy

Earl was spotting me when one of the gym employees shouted to him over the roar of the stereo speakers. "Hey, Adler! Phone!"

We had just finished up the set, so he hoisted the barbell up onto the rack and said he'd be right back. I wiped the sweat from my brow and took a couple of deep breaths while I stared up at the ceiling. Maybe I was pushing it by trying to bench 275 lbs. by my birthday.

"Vince," Earl yelled, "my wife's been in an accident! She hurt her neck. What should she do?"

"Ice it!" I shouted back. I stood up and went to the front desk. Earl handed me the phone. Although I'd lifted weights with Earl on dozens of occasions, I'd never met his wife before. People lived such separate lives, I mused.

I listened to Shirley's symptoms and told her I'd see her the next morning. Saturday mornings were my busiest. I liked working them, because I knew that I didn't have to have weekend hours and I was there because I wanted to be. Plus, I only worked until noon. That's when my weekend officially started.

I hung up the phone and headed over to the weight bench. It suddenly struck me as poignant that he'd told me his wife was on the phone—they were officially separated and going through the process of a divorce. He could have called her his ex-wife.

I didn't say anything.

The next morning, I worked on a couple dozen patients, but Shirley never showed up. I wondered what had happened. I tried calling her during the week. No one answered the phone. I tried calling her at work, and they told me she hadn't shown up.

The next time I ran into Earl at the gym, I told him that Shirley was a no-show and I was worried about her.

"She's still complaining," he said, "so I know she needs to come in to see you. Let me see what I can do."

A week passed, and finally Shirley came to see me. Enlisted in the Army as a Private, Shirley was going through alcohol- and substance-abuse counseling on base. She'd been picked arbitrarily for what victims affectionately termed the "piss test," and she'd flunked. For that reason, the medical doctor on base wouldn't treat her neck injury because the treatment would involve painkillers. Shirley wasn't allowed any drugs. Period.

She came to see me, hoping I could help her pain without drugs. Of course, I told her. That's my specialty. "But they can't know on base," she told me.

I'm not a military person. I had no idea what all the secrecy was about. But I certainly wasn't going to run to her superior and tattle. I had no idea why her urinalysis had shown traces of alcohol; all I could do was guess that drinking was how she dealt with her divorce.

A few weeks later, Shirley's name came up for a yearly physical conditioning test. Shirley told me that she needed a certain score to promote her status as Private. But Shirley wasn't anywhere near ready. Her neck was unstable and the pain was killing her. I'd gotten her to the point where she could sleep at night, but she had a long way to go. I told her that there were very few things she could do, physically, with her neck in that condition. Wasn't there something she could do about getting out of that test?

Shirley approached the physician on base to give her painkillers just to get her through the test. The physician refused, on the basis that she was still in the middle of her drug rehab program. As long as the doctor on base refused to treat her neck, the logic went, there was simply no neck problem. Therefore, she was required to go through testing.

The test consists of three simple exercises: sit-ups, push-ups and a two-mile run. The score ranges from 180-300. If you fail the test, Shirley told me, you're flagged. Literally, a cover sheet is placed on your file and it is moved to another spot. During that time, you cannot go to school, re-enlist, or anything else that means you're active. You have ninety days to retake the test. If you pass, the flag is lifted. If not, you're given another ninety days. If the injury is mild and the base physician okays it, you can substitute an activity, such as swimming or biking. For example, if you've got a cut on your hand, you can forgo push-ups but still do sit-ups. But with a neck injury, there isn't a whole lot you can do. Your body is totally dependent upon your spine and neck for any whole-body movement.

Shirley refused the test yet again, knowing that if she completed it, her neck injury would cause her a lousy score. The testers told her to take some painkillers. The whole cycle began again.

Finally, Shirley approached the Captain who was actually her boss's boss. She'd gone over her superior's head to reach the Company Commander, but she had no choice. After learning Shirley's dilemma, she received a short reprieve; the Commander waived the testing—for one month. He recommended that she receive physical therapy. The physical therapy schedule on base didn't have an open slot for two weeks. That only gave Shirley two weeks of therapy to prepare for her training.

In the meantime, Shirley continued to see me. I adjusted her neck. I gave her ice packs and ran ultrasound. I gave her mild muscle-strengthening exercises to do. We had almost completed the treatment program. Shirley was getting better. But she wasn't out of the woods yet.

The physical therapy slot came open, and Shirley kept her appointment on base. "They wanted to run ultrasound and put hot packs on me," Shirley said. "I told them that you'd already run ultrasound and that heat was bad because it would inflame the area more. It turned out that the therapist knew you. He cut me off. He said that I didn't need him."

Wouldn't you know, the Company Commander whom Shirley had petitioned caught wind of her visit to the therapist. "Since you refused the physical therapy, you must be healed. Complete your physical testing," he ordered her.

Back to square one, Shirley was discouraged, angry and disappointed. She loved the Army. She'd planned on making a career of the military. Especially now that she was going through a divorce—the Army would give her independence, travel experience, career training, a steady paycheck. What more could she want? She spent more than one tearful afternoon in my clinic bewailing her plight, but all I could do was listen. I could work on her neck, of course, but you know the old expression: The right way, the wrong way, and the Army way.

On her last visit, Shirley was withdrawn and spoke very little. Our conversation was strained. I kept my comments to a few necessary observations and instructions, and Shirley merely nodded or uttered one-word responses. Her neck had healed, but something inside of her was still broken. At first I thought she was being stoic, but then I realized that Shirley was still angry. The difference was that she had decided to do something with that anger.

Shirley applied for her discharge that day. I haven't seen her since. I know from her ex-husband that her neck never bothered her again. I know that she completed her divorce. I also know that I was impressed with her perseverance throughout her substance-abuse program. The run-around the Army gave her would have been enough to start me drinking in the first place.

CHAPTER 49

Unconventional: adj. not conventional; not bound by or conforming to convention, rule, or precedent.

The Random House College Dictionary

Bell's Palsy: a dysfunction of the 7th cranial nerve. To its victims, it can mean a slight droopiness to an eyelid, or it can signal the total loss of all nerve and muscle function on one side of the face.

When Cindy showed up in my office, I knew immediately that she had Bell's Palsy. Her body was in perfect condition, but her face exhibited all the typical signs: half-closed eyelid, limp muscles, sagging lip, drooling. She carried a tissue with her at all times and constantly patted at the saliva dripping from her mouth. She'd been diagnosed ten years before and the doctor said that nothing could be done for it. He never even recommended facial massage or vitamin B supplements.

Despite her doctor's disinterest, or maybe because of it, Cindy had tried nearly every remedy there was on her own in the past ten years. Unrelentingly, she pored through magazines, visited health food stores, consulted with health specialists. I was but another name on her ever-lengthening list.

"Have you ever tried acupuncture?" I asked her.

"No. Does it hurt?"

"It can, but in your case it shouldn't hurt at all."

"I thought it was for pain," she said. "I saw a public television special on it once."

I explained to her that acupuncture was the process of placing tiny needles at precise locations in the body to stimulate nerves. Eastern philosophy dictates that the feminine and masculine aspects of the body—the yin and the yang—can be brought back into balance with the use of acupuncture. Most western practitioners dispense with the Eastern philosophy, content to work from clinical results.

"Acupuncture is considered an experimental procedure," I told her. "Some people can undergo surgery using no anesthesia except for acupuncture. Other people receive no effect from it at all. In Minnesota, chiropractors are licensed to practice acupuncture in their offices. In Virginia, only medical doctors can perform it, and then only in a hospital setting. I have 100 more hours of acupuncture training than what is required of medical doctors in Virginia, but, because of state law, I cannot practice it and charge you for it. With that in mind, I'd like to try acupuncture on you, but I will not charge you for it."

She shrugged her shoulders. She'd been through so much already—what did it matter?

I had seen acupuncture used on Bell's Palsy before and it was extremely successful. I'd had a few unsuccessful cases. One involved a woman who panicked after the first needle was dropped. We immediately discontinued the treatment. I was excited about the prospect of helping Cindy in her quest for the normal life she had lost ten years ago. But when I'd dropped needles on all of my other patients, their symptoms had just occurred. Would I be wasting my time on a patient whose nerves had been dysfunctional for ten whole years? Better yet, why should I risk disciplinary action from the state board?

Why couldn't I practice acupuncture, anyway? I had more training than was required by state law, and I'd practiced for years, legally, in another state. Politicians. Who needed them, anyway? My patients come first. Who are politicians to tell me how to run my practice?

The treatment began. I placed several needles in Cindy's face. Occasionally, I'd twirl a needle or just turn it, to stimulate the area. I treated her twice a week and intended to follow the treatment program for a month.

Cindy came in for her fifth treatment wearing a scarf and sunglasses. Kind of an odd getup, I thought. She seemed secretive and quiet. I felt apprehensive and worried that she would drop the plan.

She sat down on the treatment table, untied the scarf from beneath her chin, and removed her sunglasses. The woman who sat before me glowed with happiness. Her grin spread from ear to ear—on both sides!

"Ohmigod!" I said. "It worked! And it only took four treatments!"

She jumped up and ran to the mirror. "I couldn't believe it, either! It was better yesterday, and today when I got up, my cheek felt all tingly and I noticed that everything could move. And, Dr. Joseph, I don't drool any more! I just can't believe it! It's been so long—I'd forgotten what I looked like!"

I called in the staff to take a look at Cindy's face. They ooohd and ahhhd and hugged and kissed her. It was like a party, and Cindy was the guest of honor.

I don't know who was happier that day—Cindy or me. Cindy, I

suppose. After all, it was her face. But no matter how many times a doctor has performed a procedure, prescribed a drug, delivered a baby, or put in stitches, there's always a chance that something will go wrong. Health care is inconsistent because patients are unpredictable. Each person who walks in the door is an entirely different individual than the person who walked in before him.

In Cindy's case, I was not only dealing with her individual physiology, but with a science that was more untested than most by Western standards. I'd had at least a half-dozen patients over the years who never responded at all to acupuncture. It wouldn't have surprised me at all if nothing had happened in Cindy's case. But I was ecstatic that something had.

Several months later, I had a patient see me after she'd twisted her ankle playing tennis. Joanne landed on the outside of her foot, nearly breaking the ankle. By the time she saw me, it was so swollen and bruised that I ached for her.

While I iced the area, I suggested acupuncture. "Will it hurt?" she asked.

"In your case, yes," I replied. "In some areas, you won't feel it at all. In other areas, particularly where you have a lot of damage, it will hurt. But the procedure is fast, and I'll get it over with as quickly as I can."

Joanne lay back on the treatment table and I began to drop needles. The first two she didn't feel at all. The third caused her to flinch. The fourth caused her to scream and nearly kick me in the face.

"Whoa!" I said, pulling her leg and foot back to the table. "Let's take it easy. Just a few more minutes." I was in luck; the needle that had caused all the trouble was still in place. I waited a few minutes, then twirled it.

"Stop it!" she yelled. "Take it out!"

I complied. She reached down and rubbed the area gently. "Ice it and keep it elevated," I told her. "I'll see you back in here in a couple of days and we'll check out the swelling."

To my surprise, Joanne showed up in the clinic the very next morning. "Dr. Joseph!" she shouted down the hallway. "Look!" She sported hot pink shorts and a plaid T-shirt. She wore new white tennis shoes with footie socks which exposed her trim ankles.

"The swelling is down! I can move my ankle!" She rotated it in all directions. "I'm playing tennis today!"

"I don't think that's a good idea," I cautioned.

"Oh, don't worry about it. I'll be fine." She skipped down the hallway like a little girl.

Whaddaya know, I thought to myself.

But I didn't really have time to worry about Joanne. I was rushing to make a flight to New York for an x-ray seminar. My head was pounding and I could feel a cold coming on. I could just imagine what the altitude would do with my eustachian tubes out of whack. The needles! I could bring my needles on the plane and use them to help my cold!

As we rocked through the thunderheads and stewardesses struggled to keep their trays upright, I concentrated on dropping needles into my hand. Despite the fact that my sinuses were plugged and my head roared with pain, the acupuncture points for a cold reside in the hand.

There, I thought to myself. All set. I'll just sit back and relax for about ten minutes and let them take effect.

"Would you like some coffee, sir?" the stewardess asked. Her eyes glued themselves to the needles sticking out of my hand. "What is that?" she said, grimacing.

"Acupuncture needles," I replied. "I've got sinus problems."

I chuckled to myself as she squinted at my nose and then looked back at my hand. I could imagine that she was wondering why I hadn't put the needles on my nose. I decided to let her wonder, and rested my head on the back of the seat. A flash of lightning caught my attention even through closed eyes. I stared out the window, but not for long. The businessman seated next to me was peering over the top of his *Wall Street Journal* and gaping at my hand.

"Acupuncture," I said, and went back to my nap.

The advanced x-ray seminar was fascinating and well worth the trip. But I did not look forward to the flight home. My cold was worse. I tossed my briefcase onto the conveyor belt at the airport security check and walked through the metal detector.

The security guard stared at the scanner intently as my briefcase ran through. She stopped the conveyor belt and stared some more. Satisfied, she sent it on its way.

"What's the problem?" I asked.

"Oh, it was just your cigarette case," she said. "It took me a minute to figure out what it was."

"Cigarette case? I don't smoke."

I popped open my briefcase and rifled through the contents. Cigarette case? "Oh," I said, "it's my acupuncture needles."

She leaned over to take a closer look. "Acupuncture needles? Neat—I've never seen them before." She sucked in her breath as I opened the lid. Rows of delicate needles lined the case, their precision reflecting in the light. I glowed with pride.

Another security guard stepped over and stared. "You can't take those on board," he said.

"Why not? They're acupuncture needles."

"According to our instructions, anything with a sharp edge is considered a weapon. That's contraband," he barked, snapping the lid shut.

"Hey, I'm a doctor. You can't take my tools away from me!'"
"Wanna make a bet? You want your pins and needles? You walk.
But you ain't goin' on that plane."
"Then wrap it up carefully and label it Handle With Care," I said.
"Yeah, yeah," he replied.

Me and my big mouth.

By the time the flight landed, my ears had popped a dozen times
and I was miserable. I wandered through the crowd gathered at the
luggage carrousel and hunted for the attendant. There she was—over
in the corner. Suddenly, she bent over and reached for something. All
I could see was her huge rear end. Suddenly, I saw her grab for
something and with a deliberate, calculating gesture, she tossed a
small box backward, over her shoulder. It arched through the air, and
before it touched the ground, I shouted, "My needles! Hey, you!"

The box landed with a thud and bounced twice. My needles, oh, my
precious needles.

I tore open the wrapping, scowling at the bright red strip of tape that
said Handle With Care, and dug for my metal case. I panicked that it
would be dented and the needles inside, crushed.

It was fine. But it wouldn't have mattered if every last needle had
been bent—either way, I was furious. "Can't you *read?*" I shouted to
the woman in the corner. My voice was lost in the flurry of activity
around the luggage carrousel. I could feel my temples pounding.
"Can't you *read!?*" I shouted again. But she couldn't hear me. As I
stared, dizzy with rage, she turned and walked away, pushing open a
door and disappearing inside.

The sign on the door read: Men's Room.

Never mind, I told myself. It's not worth it.

CHAPTER 50

The gods love the obscure and hate the obvious.

The Upanishads (800-500 B.C.)

Elizabeth had seen me several months ago for lower back pain related to shingles. She'd spent a lot of time in bed with the virus, and it took several weeks before she was back to normal. She'd had a brief bout with a pulled hamstring, too, but that didn't take too long to heal. When she showed up in my office that Wednesday afternoon several weeks later complaining of thoracic pain, I assumed that she'd thrown out her back lifting and bending. She was a secretary for a law firm and toted a lot of heavy files for the attorneys.

"I have cramps, by the way, Dr. Joseph," she said. "That may have something to do with it."

"Have you seen anyone else for this pain?" I asked.

"Yes, I've been to my family practitioner and an internist. They said I just had sore muscles."

"What kind of orthopedic tests did they do?" I asked.

"What do you mean?"

I showed her a couple of leg raises, rotations, and flexes, and explained what might happen if she had a "disc," for example. "If you move your leg this way," I explained, pulling upward, "and you felt pain here—," I paused and palpated the soft tissue in her lower back, "that would be considered a danger sign. There are hundreds of tests you can do."

"No, neither one of them even touched me. They just wrote things down."

"They didn't even take your temperature?"

"Nope."

Oh, boy. I'd have to do more of an exam than I'd anticipated.

"It's just a dull ache," she said. "It's not really anywhere that I can pinpoint."

I had her change into a gown then ran her through several orthopedic tests, and all came out normal. Nothing structural.

Then I told her to lie face down on the table. Before I even palpated her, I spotted raised, angry red spots in her lumbar region. They melded together higher up in her thoracics, creating a band across her rib cage.

"I thought your other doctors told you that your shingles was gone," I said.

"They did."

"But you said that they never touched you—they just took notes. How would they know?"

"Why are you asking?"

"Because your shingles came back," I said. "Your back is covered with a rash."

"Oh, no. I thought I was only supposed to get it once."

"Well, that's the general rule, but the human body doesn't like to follow rules. You must be under a lot of stress, and your immune system is down. You're going to have to take it easy for a while."

Elizabeth was silent during the time I took a few notes, but as I prepared to leave, she burst out, "That really makes me mad! I paid those doctors and spent a lot of time over in their offices and they both missed it! And they lied to me—they told me I could only get it once!"

"You know that the theory behind shingles is that it's simply dormant chicken pox that springs up later in life when you're under a lot of stress," I said. "It's somewhat contagious, but it's not airborne like chickenpox. If you keep the sores covered, you should be able to go to work. That is, if you can physically do so. Also, avoid contact with newborns and elderly people."

"That just makes me mad," she said. "I've had this for two weeks. I could have been putting something on it."

I had an idea. "Why don't we try ultrasound and use the gel to mix up a paste of Aspercreme and vitamin E? The ultrasound will carry it deeper into the joints."

"Sounds good to me," she said. We set her up on the equipment and I ran the ultrasound for a few minutes. Afterward, I sterilized the head. Then I adjusted her spine to ensure that there was no nerve impingement.

"I feel better already," she said. "How long will this last?"

"Anywhere from a half-hour to the rest of the day," I said. "Let me know."

She called back the next day and all but begged to come back in for an ultrasound treatment. "It got me through the day at work," she said. "It was hell last night, so all I did was lie in bed and watch TV. I wish I'd known about this the first time I had it!"

Elizabeth was so much better by the end of the week that her sores had started to scab over and she was in much better spirits. After helping her with a healthy diet and encouraging her to start an exercise program, I cut off her treatment and urged her to take more time for herself. She needed to relax and eat healthier. She lived off of coffee and often skipped breakfast.

"A virus is a strange thing," I said. "It isn't really a living thing like bacteria, so you can't kill it. You can deactivate it, and you can activate it. You can put viruses in bottles on shelves and keep them for years. You never know when they might become active again."

I didn't want to scare her, but since she'd already gotten the shingles back twice in one year, there was obviously something wrong with her immune system and her ability to cope with stress, and I needed to drive the point home. "Take care of yourself," I said.

I thought about her a lot. She was right to be angry with those doctors. How could they conduct a decent exam without ever having touched her? Why not just conduct a phone interview, in that case? Some futurists were recommending phone diagnosis via computer, but I protested that direction in health care. Sure, anyone can diagnose a cold. But what about Elizabeth's shingles? She'd never even thought to twist around and glance at her back in the mirror.

Of course, those other doctors hadn't lied to Elizabeth. They were merely operating within their scope of practice, a bunch of guys with hammers looking for a nail—but Elizabeth had been an elusive toggle bolt.

Michelle Choi fit right into that category. A nurse working in the office of an OB/GYN, she developed a sharp pain in the upper section of her lower back. She had a lot of trouble with digestion and said she felt "strange."

By the time Michelle came to my office, her menstrual cycles had been thrown off and she was very uncomfortable. She'd had a pelvic exam from her employer, who told her that he couldn't find anything wrong, but referred her to a urologist. Because she experienced burning during urination, he thought she might have kidney problems.

The urologist could find nothing wrong, but he referred her to an orthopedic surgeon. The surgeon took regular x-rays, then a CT scan of Michelle's lower back. He thought she might have a pinched nerve at L5. Nothing showed up. The surgeon referred her to a psychiatrist.

In the meantime, Michelle returned to her employer, who repeated the pelvic exam and again found nothing wrong. She told him about the psychiatric referral and he merely shrugged his shoulders.

After a year of bouncing from specialist to specialist, Michelle, anxious about seeing a psychiatrist when she believed that her physical complaints were viable, came to me as a last resort.

Since her complaints were mainly about her lower back, I examined her lower spine. I couldn't find a single thing wrong with her back. As part of a complete physical exam, I had her turn onto her back, and I palpated her abdomen. She told me about vague digestive problems, and I paid particular attention when I palpated her gallbladder. I found a nodule. When I used even the gentlest pressure, Michelle cried out in pain. There was definitely something there.

With a working diagnosis of gallstones, I referred her that day to a thoracic surgeon. His office called me back almost immediately and said that she'd been admitted to the hospital for a liver biopsy. That wasn't altogether surprising, because the liver is next to the gall bladder.

Diagnosis: Michelle had liver metastasis—cancer of the liver. She died a month later.

As a chiropractor, my specialty is orthopedics, with particular emphasis on the spine. But that doesn't mean that when an individual walks in my front door all I see is a spine made mobile by a pair of Nike tennis shoes. I see a whole person. That's what holistic medicine is all about. I'd only met Michelle once—the day I examined her in my office. But because of her history, because of the way she was batted around like a badminton birdie, particularly by her own employer, I'll never forget her plight. Hers is the type of lesson from which I will always learn.

CHAPTER 51

"Knowledge is of two kinds. We know a subject ourselves, or we know where we can find information upon it."

Samuel Johnson

When I called Mark Lane into the exam room, he looked like he'd been drugged. He was pale and anxious, and his skin was damp. He'd been referred by his family practitioner, who told me that Mark had low back pain.

After I'd taken a history, I took Mark's blood pressure. It was 198/120. Looking at the numbers, I could feel my own blood pressure rise. "Are you on blood-pressure medication?" I asked him.

"Yes. Sort of. I haven't been taking it lately."

"You really need to take it. Your blood pressure is testing high. It's dangerous not to take your medication. Do you have headaches?"

"Constantly. I can't stand the pain." Mark was also a heavy smoker—three packs a day.

I x-rayed Mark's spine and spotted an abdominal aortic aneurysm. I eyeballed it at over four centimeters, but there was magnification. It was bulging and calcified, carving away at the lumbar spine. There appeared to be an Oppenheimer's Lesion—quite rare. It didn't look good. His pain was nearly intolerable. I called a thoracic surgeon and told him to meet me at the emergency room.

"Mark," I said, "I don't want to alarm you, but I'm sending you to the emergency room. You're going to have a CT scan." He looked surprised but didn't argue. His wife had given him a ride to my clinic, and the hospital was only a half mile away, so she took him in.

The results: Mark had an abdominal aortic aneurysm that was 3.4 centimeters. I refer out anything around three centimeters for a second opinion. But this time, things didn't happen quite as I'd planned. A note arrived from the surgeon to whom I'd referred Mark. The tone was disparaging. Customarily, this surgeon cut on patients who have aneurisms that are at least five centimeters. Mark was just shy of the mark. The surgeon was upset because there was no work for him. I'd wasted his time.

Frankly, I didn't understand the surgeon's attitude. I couldn't imagine feeling disgusted that I couldn't perform a chiropractic adjustment on someone if he needed something else. The main concern was the patient's health.

Mark ended up back at the office of his family practitioner. He was given more blood pressure medication and began taking it religiously. The blood pressure went down. His headaches disappeared, as did his low back pain. The referring physician phoned me about Mark's case. "We need to monitor his aneurysm, I said. "You never know when it might act up."

"I agree," he said, adding, "Good job. I'm glad you caught it." He really lifted my spirits. He more than made up for the surgeon I'd referred Mark to. It was a happy ending, and I wasn't the least bit concerned that Mark had returned to the referring physician. I was simply happy that he was feeling better.

I was thinking about Mark when I began to hear Charlie's wails coming through the front door. He wailed in the waiting room. He wailed down the hallway. He wailed in the exam room.

I'd never met him before. His mother brought him in because her sister was one of my patients and recommended me. "Let's take a look at your leg," I suggested, toting him up on the exam table. His cheeks were stained with tears, his nose a bright cherry in the center of his face. He'd gotten past the point of crying because of the pain; now he was crying just to be crying.

I palpated his right shin and calf. He calmed. "I've been rubbing his leg all morning," his mother said, nervously playing with the buttons on her sweater. "It seems to make him feel better when I rub it. But I think it's broken. He was running around at the Dairy Queen and I wasn't watching him. Before I knew it, he'd jumped off a chair and then he just started to scream."

His ankle and foot were swollen and his two middle toes were purple. He could have broken his leg and the break was interfering with his circulation, I thought. But then, he could have damaged the foot. I examined him, then set him up for x-rays. I shot the lower leg, then the ankle, then the top of the foot.

It was a good thing I didn't place too much emphasis on the aching leg. He'd broken his ankle in two places. I showed his mother the x-ray.

"But it's his leg that hurts," she said, gaping at the viewbox.

I felt certain that if she didn't have an x-ray to stare at, she would have thought I'd made the whole thing up.

"The pain is referring up from the break," I told her. "That's actually pretty normal. I'm referring you to an orthopedist. Bones need to heal properly."

She took the x-rays with her. I received a note from her several weeks later, thanking me for my help. I really appreciate notes like that. She made my day.

It wasn't long after that when Joe, the dog trainer, showed up. This time it wasn't his lower back—it was his leg and foot. He certainly didn't jump off a chair at Dairy Queen, I thought!

"I was practicing beginning recall with a Schnauzer," he said. "I had him on lead, called him, then started to run backward so he'd follow. I didn't know that someone's kid had put a chair behind me. When I felt myself going down, I tried to catch myself, but I twisted my ankle and then I heard a 'snap.'"

I checked out his leg and foot. His toes were purple, pooled with blood. His leg appeared outwardly normal. After further examination, I x-rayed his shin, ankle and foot and thought I saw something just beneath his knee. Unfortunately, I hadn't considered that the break might be up that high, so I had the marker nearly obscuring the area.

"Have a seat, Joe," I said. "I'm going to use a tuning fork on you." A tuning fork looks pretty much like it sounds. It's a U-shaped piece of metal, about six inches long. I rapped it lightly against the outside lower part of Joe's knee. "Yee-o-o-oo-ow!" he shouted, digging his fingers into the chair.

"Bingo."

I referred Joe to an orthopedic surgeon. The break healed perfectly. And Joe learned to look behind him before he did come-forth recalls.

Nilac was brought in by her husband after she'd been to the local emergency room. She'd been in a head-on collision and was rushed by ambulance to the hospital. According to her history, she'd been thrust into the shoulder harness and was suffering excruciating pain. The emergency room physician x-rayed Nilac's chest and neck and told her that nothing was wrong. That's when Nilac's husband decided to bring her to me.

I called the emergency room and asked for the x-rays. The head nurse asked for a release. I told her I was a doctor. She refused to release them. "I don't recognize your name," she said. "Do you have staff privileges here?"

"I'm a chiropractor," I said.

"Oh. We don't release x-rays to chiropractors."

"I beg your pardon?" I said.

"We don't release x-rays to chiropractors," she repeated. "That's our policy."

"That's against the law," I said. "I'll have my attorney call you. In addition, those x-rays belong to the patient, so you must release them to her."

"No."

I'd been a guest speaker at that hospital's conference center on a half-dozen occasions. I'd visited patients there and picked up x-rays. You didn't have to have hospital privileges to pick up x-rays. Who was this person? I'd have to deal with that later, though; Nilac was in pain.

"The hospital won't release the x-rays," I told her. "It will probably take me a day or two to get through all the red tape. Meanwhile, I'm going to have to re-x-ray your neck. I hate to do that, but we don't have a choice."

"I understand," she said.

Nilac was Iranian; her father was a diplomat. She'd been brought to the U.S. as an infant and had only visited Iran once. Her hair was so black that it was almost midnight blue. Highlights reflected from the overhead lights as though they'd been painted on. Nilac's best asset was her eyes and she knew it. A Mary Kay beauty consultant, she availed herself of numerous cosmetic tricks, and I know that her beauty alone drew at least three-quarters of her clients.

I shot a standard cervical series. One of the films exposed the break in Nilac's first rib. That certainly explained the pain. It was perfectly located according to her history, too; the seat belt had done it.

"I should sue the auto manufacturer," she said. "I can't believe it!" She was normally very even-tempered, but the stress from the accident, the lack of proactive care by the hospital, and the pain made Nilac sharp around the edges.

"Not so fast," I replied. "If you hadn't been wearing your seat belt, you could have been thrown from the car and killed. I think the seat belt did a great job."

"Oh," she said, lowering her huge eyes.

Nilac signed an x-ray release form, and that evening I drove over to the hospital and demanded the x-rays. The nurse was belligerent, but I confronted her and won out. It wasn't a pretty sight, but then, ignorance usually isn't.

I returned to the clinic and immediately threw the films on my viewbox. The front shot, identical to my own, indicated nothing. The side shot, however, was out of focus. In addition, a label obscured the first rib. No wonder they didn't want me to see the films, I thought. They were too ashamed.

The next day, I sent the films to a thoracic surgeon, who said that the x-rays didn't show that severe an injury. His instructions were only to keep an eye on the patient. Without wasting any time, I returned to the hospital and showed both sets of x-rays to the head radiologist. He pondered the hospital x-rays. Then he stared at mine.

"The break happened after the accident," he said, his eyes cold and gray, shining like steel in the reflective light of the view box.

Right.

I could feel my cheeks redden as anger began to eat away at my system, working it's way up my fingertips, reaching the edges of my ears, pecking at my brain. But I refused to give in. "I don't agree. But it's not worth arguing about. I'll tell you what," I said, donning my negotiating hat, "I won't tell the patient about your x-rays. She doesn't have to know. We caught the fracture, and that's the important thing. I'm observing her. Her health hasn't really been affected."

I know that he never forgot the incident, because I never again had problems obtaining x-rays from that hospital. As far as I was concerned, we'd worked out a fair deal.

The next afternoon, I treated an eighty-year-old widow who complained that her arthritis was acting up. Edna said she felt a sharp pain on her right side just beneath her breast that bothered her when she took deep breaths. Pleurisy came to mind, but I ruled that out after I'd taken the rest of the history and examined her lungs. Her body was riddled with osteoporosis and I was sure that had something to do with it.

When I palpated the area, she cried out.

"I need x-rays," I told her.

Sure enough, when I slapped the x-ray up on the viewbox, there were breaks in her seventh and eighth ribs. "But I never fell or even bumped anything," she protested. "How could it have happened?"

"At your age, with your health history, you can break a rib just sneezing. You can roll over in your sleep and break a rib. You can yawn and stretch and break one. Even young people can break ribs from constant coughing."

I used to break ribs all the time as a kid when I had asthma attacks, I thought to myself.

She frowned, clearly puzzled. "Can you adjust it?" she asked.

"No," I said, helping her to the door, "I don't touch breaks. I'm going to refer you out. Your family doctor can tape up your ribs and give you something for the pain. Don't forget to take your calcium pills, Edna," I reminded her. "That's very important for the healing process."

The worst break I ever saw wasn't anywhere near my clinic. I was walking into a restaurant in Santa Monica when I noticed, not a half block away, a pile-up and a crowd gathering. I ran over to see what was going on and was shocked to see an off-duty police officer sprawled underneath his flipped car. The wheels were spinning like an upside-down turtle, desperately trying to right itself and looking helpless and incongruous.

The officer was screaming in pain. Gasoline spewed in all directions. He was drenched with it. The car had run into the median and flipped.

Another passerby and I helped drag the officer several feet away onto the grass, hoping we'd distanced ourselves enough in case the car burst into flames. My grasp slipped once, gasoline oozing out between my fingers. I nearly gagged on the fumes. A jagged section of bone rose from the officer's pants leg like the fin on a shark. The area was covered with exudate but very little blood. I shivered.

"My gun," he rasped. "Where's my gun? I don't want some punk killing somebody with my gun."

I turned my head to look and spotted the gun on the ground nearby. I grabbed it. "My gun," he repeated. "Give it to me." He was obviously in shock and growing delirious, and I thought it was a bad idea to give him the gun. I gave the other witness a pleading look, and he nodded. I handed him the gun. "Just hold it," I said. He nodded again.

I kneeled beside the officer and reassured him that the gun was safe. The witness held it up for him to see.

Then I lifted the officer's foot gently, elevating it so the blood wouldn't pool in his foot, although I could see that it already had. He stopped screaming as soon as I lifted it. I tried resting it on my knee, but it was too high, so I held it. "I'm holding your foot," I told him.

"My foot? Did I lose my foot? I lost my leg, dammit!" He was in shock and couldn't feel a thing, but he was tough.

"No, you didn't lose your foot or your leg," I said. "I'm elevating it. You broke your leg."

"That's all?" he said.

"You're going to be fine," I replied. I wasn't about to tell him that the bone was sticking out like an errant glacier. "The ambulance will be here any second." I had no idea if he'd be fine or not. If no one had sent for an ambulance, I could be stuck here all day elevating his leg and he'd have permanent nerve damage. But I couldn't think of anything else to say. "You're going to be fine," I repeated.

"Are you sure my gun isn't on the ground?" he asked. He was so concerned about his gun and everyone else's safety, I was awed. Had he no idea how hurt he was? The other witness periodically displayed the gun to calm the officer. After forty-five minutes, I heard a siren in the distance. Finally. My arms had begun to tremble and my muscles were burning. I couldn't hold out much longer, but his strength made me strong.

The ambulance attendants swarmed around us. "Compound fracture," I said.

"Jeez," said one of the attendants. They carefully placed him on the stretcher and I left, glancing behind me as I walked. I wondered if I'd care enough to worry about my gun if I were in that condition.

I hardly ate any lunch. I wasn't in the mood for crab legs. Every time someone at the table cracked one open, I winced. I kept thinking about that police officer and how much pain he'd be in after the surgery. But thank God for surgeons. I was right. He'd be fine.

CHAPTER 52

"Never deprive someone of hope; it might be all they have."

H. Jackson Brown Jr., *Life's Little Instruction Book*

The instructor at the postgraduate course at the Minneapolis Marriott slapped the x-ray up on the viewbox. I had no idea what it was I was looking at. It looked like a giant melted candle. A long rod, with a few divisions resembling vertebra, dripping with wax. What the hell was it? If I knew the answer, I could win a $250 subscription to a professional journal.

I could feel my jaw drop when I was finally clued in. Of course! It was so obvious! That's exactly what it looked like!

It was the tibia of a man who'd been electrocuted. The leg bone had literally melted—dripping, just like candle wax. I was truly awed.

I thought of that x-ray and felt the same awe that morning eight years later as I did a history on Al Hartman. He was a subcontractor for the local electrical company. One of his duties was to trim overhanging branches away from power lines. Al told me that his co-worker had secured a branch with rope, pulling it away from the power line, allowing them room to work. All of a sudden, the rope flipped back and smacked him, then swayed and whacked the power line. The impact sent thousands of volts straight through his body.

"I was hanging by my waist, because we always have security lines, but I was hanging backward," he told me. "The paramedics assumed that I was dead, so they just left me hanging there. I don't know how long it was—an hour? They took their time, that's for sure. I know that's where my back pain came from."

I imagined Al hanging like a half-trussed pig, belly up, arms dangling, fingers blackened, thirty feet above the safety of the ground. Al lost two fingers in the accident. There were exit marks in his neck and jaw and in the front of his thigh and shin. By the time he came to see me, Al had had so much plastic surgery that I had no idea what he originally looked like or what he might look like a year from now. His healthy skin had been used for grafting, so he had scars from head to toe.

More than anything, I was drawn to the hideous surgical job on Al's abdomen. The two burned fingers of his right hand were continually infected and regular skin grafting just didn't do the trick. What those fingers needed were living tissue—so surgeons sewed the last two fingers of his hand right onto his abdomen. He walked around with his hand in that deformed position for over a month. I couldn't help but stare at it. I tried to focus on his eyes or on my notes, but my stare kept wandering back to that grotesque surgical job. Were the surgeons on drugs? I'd never heard of such a thing.

I promised to do what I could to help him. But it wasn't going to be easy—because Al was deathly afraid of any kind of electricity, and I wanted to run interferential current on him. He wouldn't go anywhere near the equipment.

He wouldn't even flip on a light switch when he entered the room. If an assistant put him in a darkened room by accident, he'd walk right by the switch and sit in the dark.

He coped with his problem by drinking. He often showed up for his office visits drunk. I had to help him up off the table and risked throwing out my own back doing it. He spent hours down at the local bar, burning through his worker's compensation payments. He loved to play pool, somehow managed with just one arm, and was often seen leaving the bar with different women. He didn't seem to be too particular about who the women were—just so they were available. And then there was the question of his hand sutured to his belly. I'm sure Al had a hell of a time explaining *that* to his girlfriends!

It was all I could do just to get Al to show up for his visits. Eventually, I was able to adjust the cervical vertebra in his neck. And an even greater accomplishment—for both of us—was the introduction of electrical therapy. The current helped relax the muscles and speeded up the healing process. It was a great relief.

And then Al was in a car accident. He'd been drinking. I have no idea whose fault it was, but it set back his condition for months. The pain was excruciating. He dealt with it, of course, by drinking.

He became what we call a no-show. I tried to call him at home. I called his family; no one responded. I kept his file right where it belonged, just in case.

Four months after his last appointment, Al showed up at the clinic unannounced. He'd had more skin grafts. Although he was covered with scars, he was actually beginning to look human again. I was pretty impressed. But then he began to talk. I could smell the alcohol on his breath and struggled to get him out of the waiting room as quickly as possible. I brought him back to a treatment room. His eyes were bloodshot. His hair was sticking out in sixteen different directions. His untied shoelaces dragged across the carpet as he walked.

He talked about his drinking. And he talked about his women. He was obsessed with both. He wouldn't—couldn't—shut up. He wanted to sleep with every woman he saw. He couldn't get the idea out of his head.

And he'd been in another car accident. "I was pissed. I was helping my ole lady at her store, and we started to yell. We got in a big fight. I didn't give a shit what happened to me after that. So I drove my car off the road."

He hung his head, but his fists were clenched. I could see that he was still angry. His old lady was the catalyst this time. But his anger was far more deep-seated. I could see that he was angry about the electrocution; about all the surgeries; about all the pain; about losing his job; about having to rely on the government for a paycheck; about not having a normal life, a family to come home to.

As a chiropractor, I knew that I could help relieve some of Al's physical pain, but I was in no way equipped to deal with his suicidal tendencies. As gently as I could, I suggested to Al that he see a psychiatrist. I told him that another doctor could help him deal with the pain in his mind. For the first time, he admitted to me that he needed help getting over his fear of light switches. I was impressed.

Al ended up going to court for the car accident. And for his power line accident. His life seemed like it would forever consist of a series of disasters and pain and court cases, endlessly drawn out like that first jolt of electricity that ran through his body.

I wished I could find a light switch to turn off the sequence of events that started that day Al went to trim tree branches. All I could hope was that the psychiatrist Al chose could help him find his way in the dark.

CHAPTER 53

"Example is the school of mankind, and they will learn at no other."

Edmund Burke

Carol was seeing me for ptosis: droopy eyelids. She'd been to her ophthalmologist, who couldn't find the source of the problem. She'd been to a neurologist, who told her to quit wearing eye makeup. It actually wasn't a bad suggestion, since she fooled with her contact lenses and eye makeup so much that she was lucky she had any nerve endings left. But, in truth, it's more likely that a patient would get a sty than ptosis from old makeup. In desperation, she sought my help on the suggestion of a friend.

After hearing her history, it was a cinch to find her problem. Carol was a secretary at the local chapter of the NAACP and spent hours bent over a computer, straining her upper shoulders and her neck. In addition, she talked on the phone by cradling it on one shoulder with her jaw. Her sternocleidomastoid muscle—the one that sticks out of your neck when you're tensed up and that models deliberately exaggerate by tilting their heads to the side—was full of trigger points and painful to the touch. The trigger points referred pain to the orbital muscles around Carol's eyes. Carol's droopy eyelid was due to tense neck muscles.

Using trigger-point therapy based on the theory practiced by Dr. Janet Travell, an M.D. who was JFK's personal White House physician, I did a hard stretch on Carol's neck and used acupressure. It was difficult for her to relax while I bored my fingertips into her neck—it's certainly not an enjoyable procedure—but after a few days, her neck was much better and her ptosis had disappeared.

One day, as Carol grabbed her coat in the reception area, an energetic toddler yanked on the sleeve and begged for an ice cream cone. "What an adorable daughter," I praised. "What a sweetheart!" I

knew from Carol's history that she had a child, but I'd never met her.
"Oh, she's not my daughter," smiled Carol. "She's my granddaughter. My daughter is 16—this is her daughter, Sherry."

I was dumbfounded. According to Carol's history, she was only thirty-one—three years younger than I, and I'd just had my first child! I had to grab a cup of coffee. A child at fourteen years old? Carol had never married; she'd raised her daughter by herself. Her daughter was still in high school.

As I sat down in my office, staring at a pile of mail and correspondence that demanded my attention, I set down my cup and thought about little Sherry. That adorable little girl was bound to grow up in her grandmother's and mother's footsteps. She'd be pregnant in less than twelve years. I had a hard time coping with the sudden feeling of mortality that hit me when my daughter was born. I couldn't imagine what it would feel like to be a grandparent.

Angela was another one of my patients who was a grandmother before her time. She was barely forty when it happened. Angela had blonde hair that had been bleached almost white and spent so much time in the sun that her skin was leathery and dry. She seemed to enjoy the effect, and exaggerated it by wearing frosted yellow lipstick.

Angela had run away from home when she was a senior in high school in 1968. Her parents were upstanding folks, caring, intelligent. Both had college degrees, both had great careers. Angela certainly wasn't following in their footsteps—she was forging new territory. She'd gotten caught up with some wild kids in school and began to drink. From that, she moved on to grass, then LSD. She finally moved into a decrepit house on the outskirts of Houston, with a group of high school dropouts who swapped mates when they ran out of things to do.

It wasn't surprising that Angela ended up pregnant. The wonder of it was that the baby not only turned out normal physically, but also she excelled in school. Her academic record promised to take her straight to college biochem. Apparently, the child was well socialized. Someone had spent a lot of time playing with her, teaching her ABCs, helping her learn to count, showing her how tadpoles develop. Despite being ignored by a mother who had barely reached the emotional maturity of an eighth grader, others in the commune gave the child the attention and care she needed. But children aren't static. Their needs change. And when their routines change, leaving them without a safety net, they come crashing down.

Angela and her boyfriend broke up. He took off with another woman, and Angela went back to drinking. Her LSD flashbacks had tapered off, but she began using marijuana again. Eventually, Angela survived another relationship, but it only lasted five years; then her husband was killed in a freeway accident. That sent Angela into another tailspin.

By the time she met me, Angela was in a treatment program and wasn't even on speaking terms with her daughter, who had been twice arrested for prostitution, kicked out of three apartments, and beaten to a pulp by one of her boyfriends. Now she was pregnant. And the last place she wanted to go was home to mother.

No wonder Angela was seeing me for migraines. If only I could get her to quit smoking.

Angela told me the sad tale in several installments, but she hadn't the foggiest notion as to why her daughter had turned out the way she had. After all—she'd given her everything. She'd bought her all the best clothes, taken her to elegant restaurants, bought her tickets to all the latest movies, plays, circuses, skating shows and even symphonies.

In the game of life, Angela had given her daughter tons of elaborate gift wrapping, but all of Angela's boxes were empty. The gifts were merely conveniences for Angela, replacements for the tears, lack of sleep, colds, diaper changes, hugs and kisses, spankings, spilled juices, temper tantrums, homemade Valentines, scuffed tennis shoes, and first prom dresses that are all a part of the real package that is called being a parent.

Angela's daughter and new baby lived halfway across the continent. Only time would tell if distance would provide the healing necessary to keep Angela's granddaughter from continuing the pattern she had created.

But such patterns do not confine themselves to women. It takes two to make a baby. When I first met John Jeffries, he struck me as being the type of guy I could learn a lot from. Successful, good looking, a sharp dresser, he had everything going for him. He was well-respected in the community, and, everywhere he went, people knew him. After we'd met a few times for lunch and at business meetings, he started to see me in my office for sciatica.

The first thing I had him do was remove his bulging wallet from his back pocket. Most men carry their wallets in their back pants pockets, and, when they sit down, the wallets dig into the pelvic bone, pressing on the sciatic nerve. Intense pain radiates down the leg and makes life hell.

I also adjusted John's hip and ran therapy on him. He was like a new man in less than a week.

John had a real estate empire that stretched across 100 miles of prime property. He had his hands on residential and commercial property. He bought, sold and built. He even knew how to manage property once the project was completed. He did everything with gusto, including taking advantage of young women. By the time I'd met him, he was on his fourth wife.

Some guys have all the luck, people chuckled. But do they? John had married at nineteen because he had to—his girlfriend was pregnant. Four years later, he divorced and married again, this time to a seventeen-year-old. Her parents came looking for her, but by the time they found her she was eighteen, and it was too late. And the damage had already been done; John's new wife was pregnant, and the episode that followed with her parents sent the couple straight into divorce court.

Wife number three came along when John was teaching a real estate course at the local community college. She was one of his students. She bore him a beautiful son. She also bored him.

Along came wife number four. John was now fifty years old. Completely bald, his skull shone like a polished gem, and the cigar that hung from his mouth garnered more jokes and sexual innuendoes at public functions than you could imagine. Women fawned over him. He was a real life Kojak.

His wife was twenty-one. She had a college degree but had chosen to marry John and become a lady of leisure. This time, everyone said, John would settle down.

I was having lunch with a mutual friend, who had chosen this day to fill me in on all of John's personal doings. "His wife is intelligent, patient, and mature—and if push comes to shove," my friend said, dunking soda crackers into his chili, "she could make it on her own. She could be the link that would make John a stay-at-home daddy, a faithful daddy. She's a good role model for him. After all, he never had a role model growing up. You'd never know it to look at him, but he had it pretty rough."

"What was that?" I asked. "I thought he came from an upper middle class neighborhood—his dad was an attorney, and his mom was a teacher—and he had a white picket fence and a spotted dog. I swear, I heard him tell me that he had a spotted dog."

"Are you kidding?" sputtered my lunch partner. "Maybe he had a dog—I don't know. But I do know that he was illegitimate. His parents never married, of course. His mother dumped him as soon as he started to walk, and his father had no idea what to do with him, so he dropped him off at grandma's house and took off for Florida. He was raised by his grandparents."

I couldn't even finish my lunch I was so shocked. John Jeffries? Illegitimate? The missing piece was finally placed into the puzzle.

I thought that generations of unwanted children who bred generations of unwanted children were ghetto kids. They lived lives of poverty and ignorance. They had no access to information, education or money. They were welfare dependents, born in a cycle of dependency, perpetuating the cycle of dependency. Welcome to the real world, Vince, I told myself.

My instincts were right when I met John Jeffries. I knew that I could learn a lot from him. I learned that poverty and ignorance are often bred in the mind, not in the streets.

CHAPTER 54

"To live by medicine is to live horribly."

Carl von Linne

She'd been sickly all her life, she said. She'd had rheumatic fever as a very small child and ended up with a heart murmur. She'd had lots of ear infections and ended up with a 50 percent hearing loss. She wore hearing aids in both ears. She had arthritis in her joints and was taking medication for it. She had surgery for endometriosis and was on hormone therapy. She'd had her tonsils removed a couple of years ago when she tired of continuous infections. She had constant headaches and was taking Fiorinal for them. She also had asthma and allergies, particularly to cats and perfumes, and was taking shots. Despite her asthma, she smoked. She'd been given prednisone for years for her asthma, and now her system refused to produce the steroids she needed. She was forced to take steroids for the rest of her life. She was also taking high blood pressure medication.

"So what brings you into the office?" I asked. It sounded like a foolish question, considering the shape she was in. But I could tell that she'd resigned herself to leading an unhealthy life and relying on medication, so the purpose of her visit was a mystery to me. I wasn't just asking as a part of her history; I was truly baffled.

"My neck hurts."

"Where does your neck hurt?"

She pointed to the back, pretty much in the center of her neck. Her hair was cropped short, crewcut style, so I had no problem seeing the cervical vertebra protruding, particularly because she jutted out her jaw and craned her neck artificially. It looked very uncomfortable.

Her history took me over an hour. I'd never met anyone with so many problems—particularly not someone this young. I wondered how she'd made it this far in life. I motioned out her neck and found a subluxation. After I'd finished the neck exam, she shifted on the exam table and accidentally knocked her oversized, baggy leather purse to the floor. Out rolled bottle after bottle of prescriptions. Big containers. Little containers. New labels. Yellowed, peeling labels. The sound they made as they rolled on the floor reminded me of baby rattles.

She scrambled off the table and began to retrieve the prescriptions one by one, handling them as if they were gold. She zipped her purse nervously, then, with a sigh, lugged the misshapen mass over the edge of the table and dropped it on the floor. The shoulder strap hung limp, like the reins on a tired mare.

I performed a series of chiropractic and orthopedic tests. A couple of the tests indicated complications. I was concerned.

"I'm going to x-ray you," I said. "I'd like to take a look at your neck." After seeing the films, I ordered an MRI.

The films showed a moderate disc bulge, protruding chunks of calcified bone called osteophytes, and degenerative disc disease. She was a chocolate mess.

"Have you seen anyone else for your neck?" I asked. "An orthopedist, a neurologist?"

"No," she replied.

"Well, I'm going to refer you out for a second opinion. I'd like to have someone take a look at the disc I see, and the DJD—degenerative joint disease."

"What can anyone do?"

"A number of things. Traction, chiropractic adjustments, surgery."

"Can't you just give me something for it?"

Ah, the magic pill again. "I don't dispense medication," I said. "Let's wait for the second opinion."

Either Judy could walk out of my office and never come back again or I could help turn her life around. After all she'd been through, what could I do to get her to listen to me? Like millions of other people, she believed that she was stuck with her ailments forever. If a pill didn't help, then nothing would. When Olympic athletes like Mark Spitz began to show the world that asthma and other handicaps were not, in fact, handicaps but challenges, the philosophy of the medical profession began to change. It was a slow change, and it will never be complete, for medicine, by its very nature, assumes that the human body is flawed and that drugs and surgery are normal, acceptable "cures." Witness the protests from the women's movement that began in the 1960s regarding intervention during childbirth.

Intervention is the antithesis of chiropractic, which says that the human body is a perfect machine, capable of healing itself. Drugs and surgery are unusual interventions to be used only when all else fails. It is not the antibiotic which cures the disease; it is your body. The antibiotic has merely provided assistance by preventing new bacteria to reproduce. For years, surgeons removed the appendix as a matter of custom, asserting that it served no useful purpose. Somebody forgot to inform them that the healthy human body contains only necessary parts. Why would nature endow us with spare, useless parts? Small wonder then, years later, that scientists discovered that the appendix has dozens of functions just like any other organ.

Chiropractic philosophy holds that the body heals itself from the inside out. Chiropractic adjustments take pressure off of the nervous system, allowing the body to heal itself.

My patient got an MRI a couple days later. The report from the neurologist was two pages long. Eventually, the patient would need surgery, it said, but it could be forestalled indefinitely with traction.

I gave her the news. "Can't I just get a prescription?" she asked. Why she would want another drug added to the long list she was already dependent upon was beyond me.

"What you've got is structural," I told her. "We need to actually move things around—get that bulging disc back into place, make sure you don't have any subluxations. You can use drugs to kill the pain, but it won't make the problem go away."

She looked more than disappointed. She looked beaten. "I can take drugs for everything else," she said, her voice whiny, its pitch higher than normal. Stooped, pigeon-toed, hands flopping at her sides, shoulders constantly shrugging, her posture mimicked a spoiled four-year-old, but her body seemed ancient. A passerby would have guessed her to be at least seventy. She was barely forty-one.

I shook my head. Yellow nicotine stains gave her nails a rotted appearance. Tiny smoking lines indicated lips that had strained for years, pursed and taut, while lungs inhaled burning puffs of tobacco. Dark circles under her eyes were filled with fluid. She sniffed constantly.

I pride myself on my ability to help most people. I look forward to daily challenges. I relish elusive diagnoses. I thrill with the thought of helping someone out of pain with a few adjustments and a new diet. But this woman simply drained me. It was as if a dark cloud followed her everywhere. It was almost a presence I could sense. If I were superstitious, I would have said she was cursed. But I wasn't superstitious. And she wasn't cursed. She'd started out life on the wrong foot; but, after a certain point, she'd made up her mind to curse herself. She would never get better until she made up her mind that she wanted to get better. I feared that my chiropractic work would merely provide a Band Aid for her symptoms.

Nevertheless, I began a traction program. She came in three times a week, and I set her up on neck traction, adjusted her cervical vertebra, and iced the area. I was pleased that she was actually showing up for her appointments. She'd be out of pain in no time. She even smiled every now and then.

I decided to take things one at a time. Now that she was out of pain, we were ready.

"Judy, you've got to quit smoking."

She scowled at me, but I continued to talk. "Smoking increases circulatory problems and contributes to degenerative joint disease. On top of it, you've got asthma. You should know better. I'm disappointed in you."

She was clearly shocked. Appalled. No one had chastised her before for her health. She'd always been coddled. People felt sorry for her because she had so many problems. Poor Judy. Poor, poor Judy. But she was in for a surprise when she met me. It was time for her to start taking responsibility for her own health.

"Look at your nails," I said, taking her hands and stretching out her yellowed fingers. Tobacco was caked in hardened cracks. The skin was rough and calloused. "Wouldn't you like to have beautiful, long nails?"

"I've made an appointment for tips," she replied.

"I'm not talking about tips. I'm talking about your own nails. Forget the tips. Your nails are so damaged that the tips would fall right off. No sane cosmetologist would give you tips in this condition. Cut those cracked *things* off the ends of your fingers. You call those fingernails? If you quit smoking, they'll grow back better than any tips you could ever buy."

"I've tried to quit smoking," she responded nervously. "It lasted a week." She tugged at her collar, as though it were choking her.

"A week is pretty good," I said. "This time, try three weeks. It takes at least twenty-one days to create or break a habit, Judy. I'll give you one month." She appeared stunned and outraged. I'd seen business people with similar expressions who were waiting for the bus and ended up deluged with muddy water, splashed by a rushing driver.

I knew that a support group would help Judy, so I provided her with the names of two reputable groups who could help her out.

"See you next week," I said.

When I saw her next, her nails were cut short. It was like a symbol. I smiled to myself. We were on the way. Maybe I could get that black cloud to just disappear forever. What next?

"You're allergic to cats and perfume, right, Judy?"

"Right."

"Then cut with the perfume and get rid of the cat."

Her eyes widened. "You're using perfume to cover up the fact that you smell like tobacco," I said. "Once you quit smoking, you won't have to pour on perfume by the gallon. Smoking is bad for your breath, too."

She clamped shut her open mouth and looked down. "How hard

would it be for you to get rid of your cat?" I asked. "Can't you just leave it outside most of the time?"

"It's not my cat," she said. "It's my boyfriend's."

"I thought you broke up with your boyfriend."

"I did. He left the cat behind."

So you leave the cat around as a reminder, to drain yourself emotionally, I thought.

"Get rid of the cat. Take it to the SPCA. Then clean your apartment from top to bottom. Including the curtains."

She was miffed. She was steaming. How dare a chiropractor tell her how to live her life? How dare anyone tell her to quit smoking? Cut her nails? Clean her apartment?

She slammed the door behind her.

But she came back the next week. And her breath smelled antiseptic. The cheap perfume was gone. I couldn't help but smile.

"I'm so proud of you, Judy. You are doing great."

She looked surprised, then grinned. "I quit taking my allergy shots this week," she said. "I saved myself $500 dollars this coming year."

In a sense, I felt more like a football coach than a chiropractor. But it was a good feeling to be on the winning team.

I cut her visits down to once a month and called her at home every now and then to see how she was doing. I kept tabs on her smoking. She'd reduced her habit to two cigarettes a day—an immense improvement over the two packs a day she'd been burning through. I pondered her case. I normally try not to be inconsiderate of my patients' feelings. I try not to be too demanding. I know that it's hard to quit smoking, give up old habits, undergo therapy. But some people just plod along good-naturedly and take it all in stride. Others, like Judy, needed a push. Sure, I took a chance that she'd be so insulted by my statements that she'd walk out and never come back. But I figured that she was going to do that anyway. So I decided to take a chance. I was getting pretty good at reading people.

The next time Judy stopped by for a treatment, she had a gift bag with her. "This is for you, Dr. J.," she said. She held it up for me, and I rummaged through the tissue paper in search of contents.

The first thing I pulled out was a container of decaffeinated coffee. "To help you break the caffeine habit," she grinned. The second item was a package of whole wheat crackers. "Because your office staff told me that you skip meals when you get busy," she said. The last item was a Philadelphia Philharmonic Orchestra cassette. "To slow you down and relax you," she smiled.

"I'm not the only one with bad habits, you know," she explained. "Sometimes people need a push."

I could feel myself blush. Sometimes I got so involved with my patients' treatment plans that I never considered that I factored in anywhere, much less that they were observing me underneath a microscope at least as powerful as the one I was using for them. Touché, Judy, I thought, touché.

CHAPTER 55

"It is not the shilling I give you that counts, but the warmth that it carries with it from my hand."

Miguel de Unamo y Jugo

Doreen was on Medicaid. She had an adorable little daughter who talked incessantly throughout Doreen's treatments. Doreen had been laid off on disability due to ever-encroaching arthritis. After much testing, it was determined that it was rheumatoid arthritis. With chiropractic treatment, I could help her pain and keep the progression in check, but, frankly, nature gave Doreen the shaft when it came to a healthy life.

As I placed a hot pack on her lower back, I heard the distinct rumble of a stomach growling for food. It was only ten A.M. so I knew it wasn't me. Probably Doreen, I thought. She'd skipped breakfast because she was hurrying.

There it was again—but it wasn't coming from Doreen. It was her daughter, Pam. "Are you hungry, Pam?" I asked. She nodded vigorously. "Is it okay if I give Pam some r-a-i-s-i-n-s?" I spelled out for Doreen. "Sure," she laughed.

I led Pam out into the hallway and around the corner to the business office and showed her the little treasure chest we had hidden away. It was merely cardboard, painted with hinges and brackets, but to kids it was a real treasure chest. "Go ahead, open it," I urged.

She lifted the lid and her eyes sparkled with delight. Inside were dozens of little bags of toys and treats. "Take one," I said. She chose a mini-Frisbee and closed the lid.

"Pam, I thought we were going to get you something to eat. Don't you want something?"

She nodded. "Open the treasure chest."

She lifted the lid once more and spotted a little box of raisins. She looked at me for approval. "Take it," I said.

She grabbed it and skipped into the reception area. She chose a corner near the fish tank and tore open the wrapper, devouring the raisins in just a few bites. Then she opened the mini-Frisbee and tossed it from hand to hand. Even at the tender age of four, she knew better than to throw it indoors.

I finished up Doreen's treatment and escorted her to the reception area, where she donned a huge, ill-fitting winter coat. Two of the buttons were missing. She spotted Pam near the fish tank and chuckled when she saw her raisin-covered face. And then Doreen licked her lips. Hmmm, I thought. I forgot to offer Doreen something.

Next to the sign-in sheet at the front desk sat a candy dish filled with an assortment of treats. This week it had leftover Christmas candy. I pointed it out to Doreen, who gingerly picked out a mint.

"Those are getting a little old," I said. "They won't be any good next week. Why don't you just take the rest?" I grabbed a handful and stuffed them in Doreen's oversized pocket.

"See you tomorrow, Dr. J.," she smiled, and walked out the door with Pam.

When they came in the next day, I again set up Doreen on heat and electrical stim, and led Pam out to the treasure chest. "You sure liked those raisins," I grinned. "Let's see what else we can find today. But don't eat too much," I cautioned, "because it will spoil your lunch."

"No, it won't," she said with the self-assurance that only four-year-olds have. "This is my lunch."

"Right," I laughed, then remembered that her stomach had been growling yesterday in the treatment room. "Those raisins didn't spoil your lunch yesterday, did it?" I ventured.

"No lunch," she sighed, shuffling about in the treasure chest, picking and choosing among the dozens of miniature toys.

"What did you have for dinner last night?" I pushed. "A hamburger? Peanut butter and jelly?"

"No-o-o," she sighed, clearly exasperated with my ignorant adult queries. She pulled out a candy cane and more raisins, then set them side by side on the floor. "Lunch," she said, pointing to the raisins. "Supper," she pronounced, pointing to the candy cane.

She couldn't be serious. I picked her up to carry her back to the treatment room, and her ribs protruded so much that I was afraid the strength of my grip would crack them. It couldn't be, I rationalized. We galloped back to the treatment room, whinnying like horses, and galloped over to the treatment table.

"Mommy, look!" cried Pam. "Look what Dr. J. gave me!" As I removed the therapies from Doreen's back and helped her sit up, she smiled at Pam and—there it was—I know I saw her do it—she licked her lips!

"Pam," I said, stooping down to her eye level, "how would you like to go to lunch at McDonald's today?"

"Yea-a-ayyy!" she cried, leaping into the air and screeching like a spectator at a football game. "Now?"

Doreen was my last patient before lunch. "Yes, now." Doreen smiled at her daughter and said nothing. She hadn't accepted the invitation, but she hadn't demurred, either. As I escorted them out of the treatment room, I could feel the hair prickle on the back of my neck as the realization set in: Those raisins I'd given Pam yesterday had been her only meal.

"All set?" I asked, clapping my hands. "Let's go!" We all piled into my car and pulled up into the McDonald's parking lot as Pam sang nursery rhymes to herself in the back seat. I tried to keep the conversation light, but as we walked in the front door, I felt somehow as though I were attending a funeral. This would be their only meal today. Oh well, it sure beat a candy cane and raisins.

Doreen ordered a Big Mac and fries and a chocolate shake. Pam had a Happy Meal, and I had a salad and decaf coffee. Although Doreen folded her napkin in her lap, laid out her utensils with care and chewed slowly, I could tell she was starved. She was savoring every bite.

Afterward, Pam insisted on using the playground out back, so while she jumped around on the multicolored balls, slid down the slide and crawled in and out the doors and windows, I chatted with Doreen.

"Have you ever used First Call?" I asked.

"No," she replied. "What's that?" I explained to her that many communities supply food to needy people. First Call is a referral service that can help you find food from private sources. I gave her directions and she seemed pleased.

"I know it's hard for a single mother to make ends meet," I said.

"Yes," she sighed, looking at her feet. "Fred never wanted to have anything to do with me when Pam came along. He was no good."

I couldn't agree more, I thought. Then I told Doreen that she could use the local library and the unemployment office to look up jobs that wouldn't put too much strain on her joints and aggravate her arthritis. I gave her the number for a consulting firm that employed volunteers who were all retirees. They'd love to chat with Doreen, sharing ideas on ways to make money right out of her own home.

She never complained about her plight. She'd never even told me she was hungry. She loved her daughter dearly. She simply hadn't the tools to improve her lot or the motivation to do so. And she couldn't do much at all with this arthritis crippling her.

Although I had a full-time cleaning crew, I always had special needs, so I had Doreen help me out around the clinic. As long as there was no heavy lifting involved, she seemed to do just fine. A few times

I took Pam and Doreen to the grocery store and treated them to dinner in the eat-in deli bar. Afterward, we picked up a few groceries, and I carried the bags to the car. It broke my heart to think about that little girl eating candy bars for dinner. No milk. No meat. No vegetables. She was lucky she was so healthy.

But I could tell she'd gained weight. The last time I picked her up, her ribs hardly protruded at all and I really had to strain to bring her to hip level. She couldn't have gained that much weight from an occasional bag of groceries and one lunch a week at McDonalds.

I found out that Doreen was utilizing First Call, and that she'd gotten a job stuffing envelopes at home. She'd bought Pam a new pair of shoes. And then I noticed that she'd sewn shiny new buttons on her oversized winter coat. Amazing what new buttons can do, I thought. I almost thought it was a new coat.

"Thank you, Dr. J.," said Doreen, as she backed out the door, holding Pam's hand.

"No problem, Doreen. I'm glad your back is feeling better."

She shook her head, indicating that I'd misinterpreted her comment. She tried again. "Thanks. Just thank you." She smiled and walked down the hallway, keeping pace with her skipping four-year-old the whole way.

CHAPTER 56

"There is but one temple in the world, and that is the body of man. Nothing is holier than this high form. We touch heaven when we lay our hand on a human body."

Novalis (Baron Friedrich von Hardenberg)

In a world filled with microwaves, lasers, fiberoptics, liquid crystals and recombinant DNA, organ transplants and bioengineering that makes grandma a veritable bionic woman, it is refreshing to know that the human body can still function on its own. Chiropractic, a hands-on profession, helps those in pain, those who are allergic to drugs, who are too physically weak, afraid or philosophically opposed to surgery, those who don't know where else to go.

Chiropractic is the human touch that is missing in our fast-paced, technologically oriented world. *Chiro* or *cheir* is Greek for "hand." Some patients suffer from physical ailments that stem from their locked-up emotions and distorted ideas—feelings that come pouring out the moment the doctor touches them. Some people are never touched, and their chiropractors are the only human beings who have ever offered them the warmth of a human hand. It is not uncommon for such a simple gesture to unleash years of frozen pain.

Mrs. Soren was visiting me for neck pain. She'd been coming in for about a month. My working diagnosis was a cervical subluxation and stress. She had a bad habit of cradling the phone on her shoulder with her jaw. One day, as I was preparing to adjust her neck, she said, "I'm having an affair."

I took a deep breath and decided not to do the adjustment just then. I'd palpate a little more and massage the muscles. I couldn't be performing intricate adjustments and have her dropping bombshells on me.

"It started a couple months ago. We meet for lunch occasionally, and then we go to a hotel out of town where no one knows us."

I pictured a steamy scene from a B-grade movie. The image faded when I placed Mrs. Soren in the leading role. She just didn't look the part.

"My husband doesn't know. I don't think I should tell him. I don't know. Maybe I should."

It all depends upon whether or not you want to continue the affair, I thought.

I said nothing.

"I didn't intend to do it, at first. It just happened. I don't even know if I'm in love. It's screwing up my head." She let go with a loud sigh, as though a huge weight had just been lifted off of her chest. She looked up at me. I looked down at the top of her head. "Are you going to adjust my neck?" she asked. It was her way of telling me that the office visit had now returned to its normal course.

After I'd completed the adjustment, she remained on her back, staring up at the ceiling. Her hair was flattened out around her head like a halo. "Thanks for listening," she said. I left the room.

Then there was Stan. Stan wasn't a big man; he was barely 5'6". He was a wiry guy with very hairy arms. He also had a very hairy mustache. He had high blood pressure and migraine headaches. I told him to stay away from tobacco, caffeine and chocolate. I decided to wait and deal with alcohol later. Even so, he laughed at me. But he cut the items out, one by one. The alcohol came much later, but the idea of giving it up was ridiculous, as far as Stan was concerned.

"I can give up the other stuff," he snorted, "but I ain't givin' up my beer."

"Then you aren't going to get well," I replied. "We've decreased the frequency and duration of your headaches with neck adjustments and you have increased mobility in your neck. You've also eliminated some vasoconstrictors, like caffeine and tobacco. We need to work on eliminating alcohol."

"All I have is a coupla cans o' the lite stuff. It's not any big deal."

"Alcohol is contributing to your headaches," I said. "Do you like to be in pain?"

"What kinda question is that?" He was suddenly angry. "You sound like my wife. Always after me."

"It sounds like your wife cares about you," I replied.

He frowned.

"The alcohol contributes to migraine headaches. It affects the blood vessels in your head." He was silent. He crossed his arms across his chest. "Sometimes it seems like people are nagging, but they really care about you," I said. "It's hard to accept advice from people when they're telling you to stay away from things you really like."

He continued to frown. "The next time you come into my office, Stan, come in sober. If you're going to drink, you have to do it after I treat you."

His eyes widened. I could see that he thought my remark was outrageous.

I told him that in ancient times, messengers who relayed bad news to their superiors often had their throats slit after having passed on their information. "Doesn't make a whole lot of sense, does it?" I asked.

"No, it doesn't." Stan was suddenly complacent. "I shouldn't hit her."

I was shocked. I hadn't expected that. Regardless, I said, "That doesn't surprise me."

"Sometimes she just gets on my nerves. I work hard all day and I expect a little relaxation when I get home. Sometimes I just want to be left alone. Sometimes she just gets in the way."

I could feel my pulse quickening. We all want to be left alone sometimes, I thought, but we don't hit our wives because of it.

"Ya know what I mean?" he asked, looking up at me.

"No, I'm sorry, Stan. I don't. You need to talk to someone professional about it. Whatever is going on between you and your wife could be contributing to your headaches." I handed him a business card from a clinical family counselor.

He nodded. "Yeah," he sighed, "But there's nothing like hearin' that good ol' crack and feelin' like a new man. It's a whole lot easier when I can just have the doc fix my neck and make the headaches go away."

It was my turn to sigh. "Preventing them would be a better idea."

It had been two weeks since I'd worked on Cathy. She was a secretary for a law firm downtown and her neck and lower back were always bothering her because of her poor posture. Typing all day didn't do much for her wrists, either—she was showing early signs of carpal tunnel syndrome.

I called Cathy on a Tuesday. I told her that I'd missed her at her regular appointment and that I was concerned about her. She made an appointment and requested to be seen specifically by me. She sounded very tense and tired. Had she been sick? Maybe she just had cramps. I'd find out when she came in.

When I entered the treatment room, Cathy wasn't face down. I had expected her to be undergoing ice pack treatment and electrical stimulation. So, when she was sitting in a chair, staring, I knew something was up.

"You're the first person I've spoken to in two weeks," she said. Her hands were trembling. Her eyes suddenly began to fill with tears. I moved toward her, and sat on the edge of the treatment table.

"I was raped two weeks ago," she said, stifling a sob. "I was out on a date. I haven't told anyone. I haven't gone in to work. I haven't been here for my treatments. I haven't gone to the grocery store. I don't even know why I'm here right now, except that I couldn't stand it anymore."

I was speechless. I felt honored that she had chosen me to talk to, but I didn't relish the thought. The whole idea scared me. I'd never dealt with this before. I didn't know if I should touch her or stand on the other side of the room or clear my throat or just listen.

"Oh," was all I said.

She wiped her eyes with the back of her hand. I got her a tissue.

She talked for over forty-five minutes. Our office staff had codes for letting us know when other patients were waiting. If one patient was waiting, we were "down one—D1." There was a knock on the door. Clara's voice came through—"D3, Dr. Joseph."

I ignored her. Cathy continued to talk and cry. At times, she was extremely lucid, almost robotic. Other moments, she sobbed uncontrollably. She hadn't even reported it to the police. I truly was the first person she'd spoken with.

"D9, Dr. Joseph."

Cathy blew her nose. Clara slipped a note under the door. I ignored it.

"Thanks for listening," Cathy said. "Can I come back tomorrow for an adjustment?"

"Of course," I said. "I'm sure you need one." She stood to leave, and I put my hand on her shoulder. "I know some people you can talk to," I said. "They're trained to deal with this. They'll know exactly what to do and they can help you decide if you want to report it."

"D17, Dr. Joseph."

I could see that Cathy wasn't ready to call anyone else today. She'd used up all her strength just coming to the clinic and talking to me. "I'll get you some names tomorrow. Take care. Try to get some sleep."

Cathy came in the next day. She came in three times a week for the next couple weeks so I could work on her back and neck, which were injured during the rape. She had numerous bruises and muscles strains. Then I cut her down to once a week. She got the counseling I recommended and seemed to be handling everything fairly well. But I could see that it was going to be a long haul. I took a few days off, and Cathy canceled her appointments. She refused to be treated by any other doctor besides me. When I returned to the office, she came in.

"I just don't trust anyone, Dr. Joseph. I don't know how." Her eyes began to well with tears. She blinked them back.

"I'm back at work now, you know," she said, smiling. Then she looked down. "I can't let anyone else touch me. I just can't."

"You don't have to make any decisions now, Cathy," I said. "I'll be here for you. You're doing just fine."

"But I just don't know how to learn to trust anyone. I thought I could trust him. We were having a good time. I had no idea. . ."

Dealing with Cathy made me uncomfortable. I'd been robbed at gun point. I'd been beaten by gangs. I'd even been slapped by a girlfriend. I learned to distinguish between different personalities—which people could be my friends, which to stay away from. I was still making mistakes in judgment—what type of person to hire in the clinic, for example. But despite everything, I forged ahead blindly. I didn't really know how to empathize with Cathy. I felt ashamed. And I felt a little angry, too. Should I be ashamed because I'd never had something that traumatic happen to me? What kind of tricks was my mind playing on me? And how could I help Cathy?

As if reading my thoughts, she answered the question for me.

"You're the only person who's ever touched me besides my parents and a couple of boyfriends, Dr. Joseph. That makes a difference. I don't know how to explain it."

"You don't have to, Cathy," I said. "You just did."

CHAPTER 57

"I'll not listen to reason. . . .Reason always means what someone else has got to say."

Elizabeth Cleghorn Gaskell

Maureen had sprained her wrist while slamming the car door. She was a petite high school student with coal black hair and eyes that implied some Oriental heritage. I hadn't met her before and wondered how she'd heard about the clinic.

"My mother told me," she said, glancing toward the hallway. "She's parking the car." At that moment, a familiar voice in the hallway grabbed my attention like a hand around my throat, and I could feel ice crystals coagulate my blood. Sumi appeared in the doorway to the treatment room.

It had been months since I'd last seen her, and in the interim, she'd gotten a nursing degree. She allowed no introductions, and boomed her way into the room.

"I heard a 'snap' and just know that Maureen broke the wrist," said Sumi, as commanding as ever. I could sense that some of her anger was gone, but she would never give up control.

Maureen's wrist was tender and clearly out of joint, but Sumi was adamant about x-raying it. "You are going to take x-rays of her wrist," Sumi stated. "You are going to do an exam. I will look at the x-rays." She breathed in my face and tried to back me up against the wall. Even though she was a full head shorter, she was as intimidating as a 6'4" bodybuilder. But I'd dealt with her aggression before, and I could handle it again.

"It's possible that the wrist is broken," I said, "but frankly, I don't think so. The way you described the injury, it just doesn't fit. Even so, I'll x-ray it to rule out anything." I shot the films and, not surprisingly, nothing showed up. No break.

I motioned out the area and could feel the raised lunate bone on the back of Maureen's wrist. I snapped it back into place, then iced the area. Afterward, I wrapped the wrist.

"Use your other hand for awhile," I told Maureen. She was, against my best efforts, basically a bystander throughout the exam and treatment, considering the existing banter between her mother and me. "It's hard to remember, but just concentrate on picking up things with your other hand. You need to rest your wrist."

Satisfied that all was well, I bid Maureen a good day and prepared to leave the room. "I'm going to take Maureen to get a second opinion," stated Sumi. "We're going to an orthopedic surgeon."

"Why would you do a stupid thing like that?" I blurted out. "There's no break." Normally, if there is a compelling reason, I don't wait for a patient to request a second opinion—I'll encourage it. But this was different.

"Sometimes things don't show up on x-rays," retorted Sumi. "You know that as well as I."

If I'd have thought that Sumi was merely concerned about her daughter's welfare, I would have understood. But the issue dealt with Sumi's challenge to my authority. After all, we were both health-care experts. But Sumi didn't know how to read x-rays. And she didn't trust my decision.

"She couldn't have broken her wrist," I argued. "The mechanism was all wrong. She slammed the car door shut and her wrist snapped back. It was a sprain and a subluxation."

"I still want a second opinion."

You'd have thought she was going in for heart surgery or something. I was upset. And I pitied the poor M.D. who would be handling the case.

"Fine. Waste your money," I said. "Do as you please. Go ahead and take the x-rays with you."

Two days later, Maureen showed up in the clinic alone. She was carrying her x-rays.

"Dr. Joseph," she said, "I feel rotten about my mom the other day. We went to see an orthopedic surgeon, and he insisted on taking more x-rays. They were exactly the same as the ones you took. He never motioned out my wrist or said anything about icing or not using it. He was in a big hurry and I didn't like him at all. But you know what? They charged us $225 for the x-rays and office visit. And nothing was broken. Now my mom is furious that she has to pay all this money for nothing. I mean, it wasn't like you didn't warn her."

"I'm sorry about all the trouble you've been through, Maureen," I said. "I knew there was no break. Your mom saw the x-rays, but she didn't believe me. There was nothing I could do about it. You can get as many second, third, fourth and fifth opinions as you like."

"I'm embarrassed and mad."

"I know. How's your wrist?" I took off the wrap—I could see that it was a different brand than the one I'd put on her—and I could see that her wrist was almost as good as new. "Keep resting it," I told her. "And don't worry about your mom. Those things happen. I'm sure she was just worried about you."

Maureen's frown and lowered gaze told me that she believed that about as much as I did. "Thanks for coming by, though," I said. "Stay away from car doors." She smiled and left.

That was nice, I thought. She didn't really have to come in and tell me that. Besides, I had more than my share of argumentative patients, so Maureen's mother wasn't going to cause me to lose any sleep.

Dolores Pastry, on the other hand, caused me to lose a lot of sleep. She came in one day with complaints about neck pain, back pain, shoulder pain, leg pain and headaches. She had a history of sciatica, lupus, alcoholism and cancer. She was forever ill, and when she wasn't in bed with an illness, she made one up.

Her neck pain stemmed from a small bone spur. I helped relieve the pressure and pain with traction and adjustments. The bone spur was causing arm and hand pain, and I was hoping to catch it before she ended up with drop attack—she could start losing neurological input and drop objects, such as a pen or a cup of coffee. If she started to lose her grasp, she'd definitely be getting worse and might need surgery.

But Dolores hated neck adjustments. The traction she didn't mind, except that it took so long. She would much rather have taken a magic pill and waltzed out the door.

Considering the fact that she was still drinking, there wasn't a whole lot I could do about her holistically. She certainly had enough illnesses to keep me working on her indefinitely, but I felt that we would have made more progress if she'd chosen a drug and alcohol treatment program.

Her case was frustrating not only because it was difficult to determine where to begin with such a litany of illnesses, but, in addition, she lied to me about her drinking. She told me that she never drank at home. Not more than five minutes later, she told me that her brother had come over to visit and they'd had a couple of gin and tonics together. I had also run into her at a couple of parties and she was, as they say, three sheets to the wind. I wondered what else she was lying to me about.

I had her on a program of adjustments for her lower back but she gave up on that because she couldn't keep the appointments—she'd cancel at the last minute or sometimes not show up at all.

She responded best to her thoracic adjustments. She sometimes exhibited upper back pain, particularly behind her shoulder blade, and those episodes were relieved instantly with an adjustment. I was right.

She was in this for a quick fix.

I tried to explain to her just what sort of shape she was in and what it would take to get her well, or at least out of pain. She wanted nothing to do with it.

After she'd missed two weeks' worth of appointments, I had a staff member call her at home. Her husband answered the phone.

"Oh, didn't you know?" he said. "She's having surgery tomorrow. She's having the bone spur removed from her neck. She said she couldn't stand the pain any more."

My heart sank when I heard the news. A quick fix. She'd spent years abusing her body, and now she wanted an instant cure from a scalpel. I called her husband personally.

"Was she dropping things?" I asked.

"No," responded her husband. "Why?"

"It's a symptom to look for with her particular problem."

"Actually, her pain got better when she was seeing you," he said. "I don't know why she quit."

After two more weeks, I called Dolores at home. Her husband answered and said she was resting in her bed upstairs. "How is she feeling?" I asked. "How did the surgery go?"

"Well," he paused, choosing his words carefully, "she's in a lot of pain, what with the surgery and all. I suspect she'll be feeling better in a few days."

"What about her arm pain?" I asked. "Is that better?"

"I don't know," he said. "I didn't ask her."

"Well, I'll check back later," I said. "Please tell her I called."

I was upset. She hadn't even called to request her records. I hoped that her surgeon had enough information. Assuming he did, my x-rays and records may have helped, anyway. I always felt more comfortable when I could collaborate on patient treatment.

It wasn't more than a week later that I ran into Sally Mercer at my Rotary breakfast. "You're looking a little down," she commented. "What's the problem?"

Without using her name or going into specifics, I briefly outlined Dolores' plight and told Sally how much it bothered me. I realized that I couldn't help everyone, but when people chose to destroy themselves through some unconscious desire, it ate me up inside.

Sally was the administrator for a brand new nursing home that had been built entirely from the private donations of one individual. The architectural design had won three local awards and was up for national competition.

"I'm afraid I don't know all our patients by name," Sally commented, "but something about your patient sounds familiar. Her name wouldn't be Dolores, would it?"

I jerked my head around and held my breath. "How do you know her?" I said, but even as the words came out of my mouth, I knew.

"She was just admitted into our long-term care program yesterday," Sally said. "She had a stroke and she's totally paralyzed from the neck down. She'd just had surgery no more than two weeks ago. What a shame. She was only sixty years old and she still played golf until last month."

"What made you remember her name?" I asked.

"Her husband is suing the surgeon and the hospital," Sally said. "He thinks that the stroke was caused by the surgery. I heard that she had quite a history, so it's going to be a bit difficult to prove. Certainly, her physician would have documented everything carefully and wouldn't leave himself open."

My mind focused in on the pages and pages of history I had on Dolores. Could that information have prevented the surgery? I sighed. It certainly wouldn't do anyone any good now.

Later that day, I found a note on my desk from Clara. It was a message from a local attorney informing me that I was about to be subpoenaed for Dolores' files. For some reason, Mr. Spock's famous Vulcan quip echoed in my mind: "Fascinating." I felt detached and without emotion, but certainly not without curiosity. I would never have thought it could have ended up this way.

Soon after, I was asked to give a deposition. An attorney and court reporter came to my office and I gave them the run-down on Dolores. Although my comments were professional and specific, and I knew my adjustments had helped, I worried that Dolores' alcoholism would blow the case.

I was wrong. The hospital and physician agreed to settle out of court. Dolores and her husband were awarded $1 million. It was a bittersweet victory.

The sad thing about it was that although a surgeon used poor judgment taking on Dolores' case, it was Dolores herself who had started the whole thing. She wanted a quick fix. A magic pill. Instant gratification. She wanted no part in her own recovery. She would place the entire responsibility in someone else's hands, regardless of the outcome.

Gary was another example of refusing to face reality. The moment he walked into my office, I recognized the mask of Parkinson's. His face was stiff and expressionless, just like a mask. He also exhibited classic Parkinson's finger roll—where the center finger and thumb click together, nervously playing an invisible castanet.

Gary came to me filled with pain, rigid, stiff and tired. His joints seemed like they'd been soldered together. He'd been to two orthopedic surgeons, a family practitioner, and a neurologist. All had diagnosed him with diabetes. Two had told him he had Parkinson's syndrome. Gary was on medication for his diabetes but wasn't excited about taking it. He took it when he felt like it. Which was about once a week. If he remembered.

I had sent Gary out for lab work and the results showed that his blood level was totally skewed and he was very obviously diabetic. I encouraged him to take his insulin. He of course ignored my advice.

I took several x-rays. What I saw when I looked up at the view box was totally unexpected. I thought that he had the beginning stages of arthritis, but he had a classic case of DISH—Diffuse Idiopathic Systemic Hypertrophy. His spine was fusing together.

I was furious. How could so many doctors have missed this? It was right in front of their noses. Were they blind? Gary had been bouncing around from doctor to doctor, seeking a diagnosis, praying for a cure, and the whole time it was right underneath everyone's nose.

Diabetes is commonly found in people with DISH, I reminded myself. If there were any doubt in my mind from the x-rays, the diabetes would be another clue.

But my anger toward the other doctors was quickly spent. When I called Gary into my office that Monday and explained the disease to him, he instantly jumped into denial.

"I've got Parkinson-like symptoms," he said. "We can work on those."

"You don't understand," I persisted. "This is a serious disease. I can help loosen up your joints and I can recommend a diet that will help you stay healthy. I'm also going to order a CT scan for you." I knew that Gary had DISH. I knew that he had diabetes. The Parkinsonism I wasn't convinced of. I was concerned about calcification of the posterior longitudinal ligament but couldn't find any references for it, so I called a specialist in Minnesota. He agreed that the premise should be investigated.

But Gary had an even simpler solution: he quit seeing me. I found out from his sister that he'd visited with a psychic and a homeopathic physician. They'd both agreed to treat his "Parkinson-like symptoms." Never mind that they'd never even heard of DISH. Gary was being told what he wanted to hear.

He showed up in my clinic a year later asking for an adjustment. He told me that he was pleased with the work his psychic was doing; she convinced him that his problems stemmed from a past life and all he had to do was work through it all.

"I can certainly do the adjustments, Gary," I said, "but you've got to get out of this denial. You don't have 'Parkinson-like symptoms,' you have DISH and diabetes. You need to take your medication." I recommended a Parkinson's support group. He expressed minimal interest, but I found out that he'd finally attended a few sessions. I gave him as much material as I could find on DISH and Parkinson's. I copied pages from books. I loaned him cassettes. He digested the information like a starving beast, but it failed to nourish him.

His joints were so jammed by this time that adjusting him was like trying to pry rusty lug nuts off of an old flat tire. I was sweating by the time I'd finished. And I wasn't altogether certain that it had all been from physical exertion.

"Why did you come back?" I asked.

"Because I was in pain. My joints hurt. I wanted adjustments."

"That's only treating your symptoms, you know. I told you the truth and those other people—that homeopathic physician and psychic healer—didn't, you know. They told you what you wanted to hear. Homeopathic remedies are great. I use some of the remedies for myself because they don't have as many side effects as drugs, especially with all my allergies. But I can guarantee you that neither one of those people has ever heard of DISH."

My little lectures were wasted. Gary never made another appointment. He even quit seeing the homeopathic physician. He quit taking all his homeopathic remedies, all his insulin, all his blood pressure medication, and relied solely on the psychic. He told me that the psychic was helping him more evenly distribute his life forces, his energies. He was not balanced. All he needed to do was meditate, relax and travel back in time.

Gary's hypertension was getting worse, and he wasn't doing anything about it. He refused my adjustments, refused his medication, and relied on his psychic healer. One month later, he died of a heart attack. He was forty-one years old.

Although I expected the news, it still shook me up. Eventually, he would have died anyway, I rationalized. But I could have helped him relieve much of his pain. His medications could have helped his hypertension. He could have lived much, much longer. He could have done this, he could have done that. . .what did it matter now? I'd fed him with pages and pages of information. I'd instructed him for hours regarding diet, exercise, and details of his diseases.

But I'd made a fatal mistake: I'd appealed to Gary's intellect, totally ignoring the power of his denial. It was Hitler who said "I use emotion for the many and reserve reason for the few." Gary's modus operandi was emotion. I'd fed him pages and pages of material that dealt with his diseases on a purely intellectual basis, when, all along, he'd been craving food for his soul. I hadn't even come close.

Losing a patient to death is like losing a body part. It's traumatic. It's devastating. It's shocking. But life goes on. You learn to work around the missing part, but you never forget what was once there.

CHAPTER 58

"To be ignorant of one's ignorance is the malady of the ignorant."

Amos Bronson Alcott

My introduction to Alexander came in the form of a spinal exam. Since his mother, Lisa, had severe scoliosis and received weekly adjustments, she was worried that Alexander might have inherited the same disorder. Lisa's spine was supported with a rod, and I adjusted the vertebra above and below the rod. Alexander's spine seemed normal during the exam, but Lisa and I agreed that he should be checked every six months. He seemed like a perfectly normal kid.

One morning Lisa showed up in my office clearly shaken. Her eyes were rimmed in red and, as soon as I closed the door to the treatment room, she began to cry.

"Dr. Joseph, they're going to take Alexander out of school. They say he's learning-disabled. They can't handle him and he's not paying attention in class."

"What sort of tests have they done?" I asked.

"Tests? They haven't done any yet. All I know is that his teacher says that she can't handle him. He ignores her when she's trying to explain things, and then later he'll lose his temper and start to cry over the littlest thing. He's been pretty wild at home, too. He throws temper tantrums and sasses back and I don't know what's wrong with him. I thought we finished with this stage after he was out of diapers, but ten is much too old! He just can't seem to remember the meaning of the word 'no.'"

Lisa blotted the corners of her eyes with a tissue and said, "They want to put him on Ritalin."

That caught my attention! Ritalin was this decade's fad drug for this decade's fad disease. In the '70s and '80s we'd been through Legionnaire's Disease, Toxic Shock Syndrome, and the Yuppie Flu.

How simple to find a problem like Attention Deficit Disorder so that you can pop your kids full of drugs and send them back to school—easy for Mom and Dad, easy for the doctor. I'd met dozens of parents who were never warned about the side effects of Ritalin and were just now beginning to pay the price—children who were permanently learning-disabled, whose growth was stunted, who had been cheated out of a healthy life. Many children had doctors who failed to do proper exams and research, considering alternatives such as new diets or lifestyle, not to mention preventative measures. They simply took the word of school nurses, teachers and parents. The whole idea made me shudder. Sure, there's a place for Ritalin. But who's doing the diagnosis and determining need?

"Who diagnosed him?" I asked. Lisa shook her head. She knew enough about Ritalin and its side effects to know that she'd try anything else first. I suggested that she go back to school and find out what sort of testing was done. Then she could find out if Alexander's teacher had any special skills to recognize or handle LD kids.

A week later, Lisa was back for her adjustment and filled me in. "The school tested Alexander," she sniffed, "and he failed the tests. He's way behind his age level in motor control and math and everything. I just don't understand it. Just six months ago, he was doing fine. The school's test backed up what Alexander's teacher said. But I think she just doesn't like him. She never liked him from the start. I don't think the system is objective."

Lisa was beyond tears and beginning to shore up her spirits. She had a self-righteous streak that sometimes came in handy. "The teacher said that Alexander could not function at all unless I put him on Ritalin. She refused to have him in her class otherwise! I feel like I'm being blackmailed. The other classes in his age group are full. So I'd have to take him out of school altogether. We can't afford a special program or private school."

"Let me take a look at him," I offered. "Maybe I could find something they missed." She brightened and promised to bring him in.

Alexander did seem changed. Since it had been six months, I did a scoliosis exam and his curve seemed fine. He fidgeted during the exam, wiggling, coughing for no good reason, and scratching himself when he didn't really itch. His hands were shaking.

"What sort of a diet does Alexander have?" I asked. The reply was typical: hot dogs, hamburgers, pizza, macaroni, fried chicken. What about desserts? And drinks?

"He loves chocolate and Coke," Lisa said. "He needs his daily fix." She grinned at Alexander and he rolled his eyes.

"Do you know how much caffeine is in chocolate and Coke and other cola drinks?" I asked Alexander. "You're going to stop eating chocolate and drinking Coke and then you'll get good grades in school and you'll grow up to be a football player," I suggested. "Would you like that?"

Alexander eyed me suspiciously and said nothing.

"I'd also like Alexander to take vitamin C every day," I told Lisa. "He needs to boost his immune system." I paused for a moment, pondering an idea. Lisa was a clever woman. And she cared deeply for her son. I decided to try out the idea.

"Wouldn't it be interesting," I said, scratching my chin and staring out the window, as though deep in thought, "to see what they'd say if you sent Alexander to school with vitamin C instead of Ritalin?"

Lisa took the bait. Her blue eyes twinkled and she smiled mischievously. "I could send him to school with the vitamins, with instructions to take one every four hours. The teacher wouldn't know the difference between that and Ritalin."

The ploy didn't bother me in the least, since Alexander had never been diagnosed by an M.D. Teachers can recognize all sorts of symptoms, but that doesn't mean they can diagnose, or prescribe drugs, for that matter. The whole thing made my blood pressure rise. Besides, if the diet changes, adjustments, and vitamin C didn't work, we could say we'd tried everything. Then Lisa would be able to accept the Ritalin and not lose any more sleep over it.

I started Alexander on a treatment plan of full spine adjustments, cervical (neck) adjustments and some cranial work, which meant that I worked on the muscles on his head and neck, focusing on acupressure points. Most healthy kids don't need too many adjustments, but Alexander's joints all needed adjusting.

I also told Lisa that some people are sensitive to fluorescent lighting and that full-spectrum lighting often helps in that regard. It helps plants grow that would otherwise wilt unless they had real sunlight. Although it's more expensive than fluorescent lighting as far as initial cash outlay, they last longer, so the investment makes up for itself.

Two weeks later, Lisa gave me a progress report while Alexander read in the reception area. "He's so much calmer, Dr. Joseph," Lisa said. "He listens to me when I talk and he doesn't fidget so much. He really used to be a discipline problem, and I didn't realize how bad it was until he started to behave. What a contrast. He's off caffeine, unless someone sneaks it to him at school, and he doesn't even miss his chocolate because I've given him carob and tried new things like strawberries and cinnamon. I'm surprised it's been so easy. . .well, for the most part. The first couple days were awful. He threw something at me and slammed a door in my face, but I expected that." Her eyes widened and she leaned forward.

"The teacher accepted the vitamin C without question. Can you believe that?"

"Do you feel comfortable with what you're doing?" I asked.

"You bet. I know that teacher doesn't like him and I'm going to prove it."

"What happens when he has caffeine? Can you notice a difference?"

"Yes! I was shocked! It's like night and day. I am so relieved. I'm convinced that's it. And I know the adjustments help, too."

"Let's give it three months, Lisa," I said. "This could be a fluke. He's almost an adolescent and he's going through all sorts of changes. You can't draw a permanent conclusion after just two weeks. Okay?"

"Okay."

Some kids digest chocolate and caffeinated drinks with no problem. Their metabolisms just send the stuff on through. But other kids—not to mention adults—cannot tolerate the least bit of caffeine without turning into monsters. Headaches and other illnesses follow and, by then, it's extremely difficult to find out what caused it all. Alexander had that type of metabolism. I was relieved that he was old enough to comprehend the "why's" of giving up his favorite treats and beverages. Much younger children beg and whine and feel like we grownups are just trying to be mean.

After three months of marked improvement on Alexander's part, Lisa squared her shoulders and arranged a meeting between herself, Alexander, his teacher, and the school principal. Victorious, she strode into my office glowing with pride and relief. She was bursting to tell me what happened.

"I asked the teacher to tell the principal if Alexander's behavior had improved over the past three months," she began. "The teacher said, point blank, that since Alexander had been taking his 'Ritalin,' his behavior was 100 percent better and he was much easier to handle in the classroom. On top of it, his test scores are back up to where they're supposed to be."

Lisa smiled and sighed, then continued. "Then I said I was going to take Alexander off of the 'Ritalin.' The teacher adamantly refused to accept him in her classroom if I took him off the drug. Then I told the principal that I thought Alexander's teacher was prejudiced against him, that she had mislabeled his learning disability and that I could prove it. The principal said, 'How can you prove it?' and I told him about the vitamin C, taking Alex off caffeine, and getting chiropractic adjustments.

"The teacher's jaw dropped. Her face was bright red. I gave them your phone number, by the way, in case they want to talk to you. Anyway, the principal agreed to place Alexander in another classroom with another teacher, so he's mainstreamed again! I also told them about full-spectrum lighting and the principal said he'd look into it."

It's the Lisas and Alexanders of the world that make me look forward to getting up in the morning. Looking back on the numerous trips I made to the hospital as a child, the dozens of times I was poked with needles, infused with epinephrine, made to breathe a distasteful solution of moist, salty oxygen, I can't help but wish I'd known about chiropractic. Yes, my grandfather took me to a chiropractor to relieve my aching neck and shoulders as a paper boy, but chiropractic as a health profession meant nothing to me. My world consisted of long days spent studying in my sterilized room, subsisting on Tedrol (a depressant), gazing out the window, wishing I could be out there playing. In high school, I reached my adult height of six feet. But my weight was a mere 100 pounds.

Ironically, it is because of the way I misspent my youth that my fervor for chiropractic continues to burn. I cannot bring back my sequestered afternoons in my bedroom, yearning for cats and dogs and plants and impassioned games of Kick the Can in dusty parking lots. But I can guide today's children toward a more healthy lifestyle with chiropractic adjustments, dietary advice, exercise plans, enthusiasm and hope.

Drugs are a last resort and must be used carefully. Too many patients and physicians use them carelessly as medical brooms to sweep the dust under the rug. You've only got one body, and it's designed more perfectly than any computer ever devised. Auto accidents and gunshot wounds aside, it shouldn't be necessary to use invasive techniques to keep that human computer running smoothly. I'm working to ensure that those stuffy afternoons getting a mindless, quick fix in Dr. Murphy's office have been erased from our health-care system forever.

EPILOGUE

"The doctor of the future will give no medicine, but will interest his patients in the care of the human frame, in diet, and in the cause and prevention of disease."

—Thomas Edison

The past few generations have grown to accept, expect, and demand services, commodities and technology that once were considered not only impossible, but laughable. Flight. Heart transplants. Space exploration. Recombinant DNA gene splicing. Cloning. Fiber optics. Our craving for instant gratification has created a frenzied, insatiable appetite for fast food, drive-up technology, and doc-in-the-box health care.

We've gorged ourselves on knowledge, in the process becoming technological vampires, sucking the blood of industry and leaving behind a meaningless shell of humanity. Without tempering knowledge with wisdom, we risk spinning backward into the past, to a time when brute force was a given and compassion, creativity, and culture were bourgeois luxuries.

The finely honed skill of surgery has saved millions of lives and helped alleviate suffering in millions more. But because of the lure of its relative safety and its appeal to those who seek instant gratification, unnecessary surgery has also killed millions and crippled millions more.

The proliferation of prescription drugs has diminished much suffering and helped bring millions of people back to health. But it has also exploded into a billion-dollar stock market industry, at the same time providing a dangerous panacea for ignorant patients and overworked or incompetent doctors. "Take two aspirin and call me in the morning" has metamorphosed from a lighthearted cliché to a cynical commentary on a calloused medical profession.

We have come to rely so much on technology, on drugs, on miracle cures that we have become inured to the reasons we need such things in the first place. We refuse to accept responsibility for our actions, then blame the health-care system and the government for not curing us.

"First, do no harm" is the most important part of my philosophy. I have no desire to run elaborate experiments at the expense of an innocent victim. My goal is not to impress patients with bells and whistles; it's simply to help them help themselves. The fact that no diagnosis would ever be complete unless I touch the patient keeps me in touch with my own philosophy and goals.

I have a compulsion to treat as many people as I can. I have a craving to help people. I think it makes me feel as good as my patients feel. I push myself too hard sometimes, to the point of physical exhaustion. Several classmates of mine, particularly women, found it necessary to take up weight lifting to ensure them the strength for adjustments. Every profession has its unique form of physical stress. Surgeons, OB/GYNs, dentists who are on their feet all day constantly stress their backs. Chiropractors have physical stress in addition to the emotional and spiritual stress that comes from close physical contact with patients on a daily basis.

Some people believe that a form of spiritual energy can actually be transferred from one individual to another. Kirlian photography purports to prove such a theory. I have seen no proof of such a transference, but I like to keep an open mind. I do know that living creatures, particularly primates, need touch. Researchers have experimented with baby chimpanzees, separating them from their mothers at birth. Consequent infant chimp deaths were documented as being attributed directly to deprivation of physical contact. Whether the need for contact is purely emotional or something physical, stemming from electrical energy, heat or something else altogether, remains to be seen. But the fact remains that touch is necessary.

In this world where the miracle of technology is too often abused, I have chosen a form of healing where the human body itself is instrumental to the healing process. It's that simple.

Vincent Joseph, D.C.

Hampton Roads publishes a variety of books on metaphysical, spiritual, health-related, and general interest subjects. Would you like to be notified as we publish new books in your area of interest? If you would like a copy of our latest catalog, just call toll-free, (800) 766-8009, or send your name and address to:

Hampton Roads Publishing Company, Inc.
891 Norfolk Square
Norfolk, VA 23502